START SMALL, LIVE BIG

Thrive Through Change To Live The Life Of Your Dreams

*Lisbeth,
You are so awesome!
Live Big!
♡ Betsy*

BETSY PAKE

BALBOA
PRESS
A DIVISION OF HAY HOUSE

Copyright © 2017 Betsy Pake.

All rights reserved. No part of this book may be used or reproduced by any means, graphic, electronic, or mechanical, including photocopying, recording, taping or by any information storage retrieval system without the written permission of the author except in the case of brief quotations embodied in critical articles and reviews.

Balboa Press books may be ordered through booksellers or by contacting:

Balboa Press
A Division of Hay House
1663 Liberty Drive
Bloomington, IN 47403
www.balboapress.com
1 (877) 407-4847

Because of the dynamic nature of the Internet, any web addresses or links contained in this book may have changed since publication and may no longer be valid. The views expressed in this work are solely those of the author and do not necessarily reflect the views of the publisher, and the publisher hereby disclaims any responsibility for them.

The author of this book does not dispense medical advice or prescribe the use of any technique as a form of treatment for physical, emotional, or medical problems without the advice of a physician, either directly or indirectly. The intent of the author is only to offer information of a general nature to help you in your quest for emotional and spiritual well-being. In the event you use any of the information in this book for yourself, which is your constitutional right, the author and the publisher assume no responsibility for your actions.

Any people depicted in stock imagery provided by Thinkstock are models, and such images are being used for illustrative purposes only.
Certain stock imagery © Thinkstock.

Print information available on the last page.

ISBN: 978-1-5043-7051-6 (sc)
ISBN: 978-1-5043-7064-6 (e)

Balboa Press rev. date: 12/16/2016

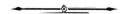

This book is dedicated to Craig, who lovingly and haphazardly believes I can do anything. For everyone reading who knows there is a Big Life waiting for them and aren't afraid to take the risks to find it and for Duane and Kim who encouraged me to take the risk to find mine.

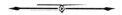

CONTENTS

Foreword ix
Introduction xi
Chapter 1   Creating Your Vision 1
Chapter 2   Know What You Believe 13
Chapter 3   C.H.A.S.E. Your Big Life 25
Chapter 4   At All Costs 38
Chapter 5   Finding Your Passion 45
Chapter 6   Balanced Health For Living Big 52
Chapter 7   The Value of True Connection 66
Chapter 8   Our Common Thread 73
Chapter 9   The Big Kahuna 78
Chapter 10   The Power of Starting Small 85

FOREWORD

After my presentation on thriving through change, many are baffled. Rising from dire poverty in a tiny Haitian village to being a famed motivational speaker is inconceivable to them. Others think I'm lucky or I have some a secret.

The reality is, I'm not lucky nor do I have a secret. I suppose if there's a secret to my success, it's within this book. It's the message Betsy Pake is sharing with the world. Start small. Live big. As Christopher Morley reminded us, "Big shots are just little shots that keep shooting."

Most people see the big shots on television or at the top of their games. They assume it has something to do with luck. The reality is, the vast majority of people you see at the top started at the bottom. In fact, there's no top without a bottom. You can only climb from the bottom. The top comedians and singers you see out there started performing in obscure little pubs for free. Every big business was at one time a small business.

The sad thing is, most people chase success the wrong way. Somehow, the clues are invisible to them. They see others living big.

They feel discouraged. They wonder why they are struggling while others are so prosperous.

If that's you, please do not be discouraged. Do not compare yourself with others. It's okay to be where you are on your journey. Those you admire at the top were exactly in your position at one time. Instead, create your success by focusing on your next step.

There's nothing wrong with you. There's nothing missing. You may need to pivot. But, don't give up. Fortunately, Betsy lays out a proven framework that can help you speed up the process and skyrocket your results faster. She shares with you the exact step-by-step formula in this book.

When I arrived in this country broke, clueless, and unable to speak any English, Start Small Live Big is the kind of book I wish I had at my disposal. I'm excited you are about to read it. I strongly suggest you get a copy for your friends and family members; especially those who tend to have a negative attitude.

Finally, I want to remind you any dream that is worth chasing is worth starting small. Don't wait for the big break or for all your ducks to be in a row. That can lead to unnecessary frustrations. Start now. Start small. Start where you are.

Keep pressing on even when the results are not coming fast enough!

Rene Godefroy
Legendary Motivational Speaker
Bestselling author of
Kick Your Excuses Goodbye

INTRODUCTION

If you want more out of your life, this book is for you. You may want increased happiness in your relationships, more robust careers doing work that you love, or you may want to rebound from failure and let-down while focusing on the things that are most important to you, your families, and friends.

In today's culture of "Go Big or Go Home," it's easy to forget that big things started out small. The messages we receive every day from the media can make us feel as if we aren't doing enough, and that we probably can't progress to living the life we wish we had.

We may feel focused for a short time, working on our career or our health, but then slide back into what we know and what is comfortable. We want to make changes, but it seems like change can be too difficult to maintain.

A few years ago, my then preteen daughter was experiencing a lot of anxiety. She would freeze and have trouble controlling her breath. We went to doctor after doctor, and one finally explained it to her by saying that she had an army in her brain that was very strong. Stronger than it needed to be and that we needed to teach her brain that she was safe.

I was curious about this, did my own research, and discovered that the amygdala, a limbic system structure that is located deep within the temporal lobes of the brain and is involved in many of our emotions, especially those that are related to survival, was at the core of her anxiety. Your amygdala controls your "freeze, fight, or flight" response, and with my daughter, it was in overdrive. When this happened, the front cortex of her brain shut off and she no longer had access to rational thought or problem solving.

At this time, I was working one on one with my coaching clients. There were times when I would ask them to do something out of the ordinary, and I would see a response in them that I recognized as similar to my daughter's. They didn't have anxiety attacks, but they felt a resistance they couldn't quite understand or explain.

I decided to work with them using the same methods I had used with my daughter. We broke big steps into small chunks and worked with those small chunks until they could be achieved. With this method, we could essentially tip-toe right past the sleeping amygdala and push the threshold of what they could do further and further, until soon they were accomplishing things they hadn't been able to do before. These new actions and small successes bred more motivation, and soon my clients were pushing past obstacles they hadn't been able to overcome in the past.

You may struggle with figuring out where to make change in your life right now. It may seem like life isn't going your way, but you aren't exactly sure what you would change. Or perhaps you are aware of some changes you need to make in a few areas of your life, but you've just never been able to get moving to figure out the steps to make real change happen.

By implementing my C.H.A.S.E. framework I teach in this book, I've seen people get extreme clarity on areas of their lives in which they were unsatisfied. They were able to lay out a path they could follow step by step in order to achieve success.

I promise if you follow the steps I outline, you will begin to develop a roadmap. If you take the time to examine the areas of your life I discuss in the pages ahead and map out your small steps, you will begin to find renewed motivation, feel energized, and see the success that has eluded you in the past. You will understand what has been holding you back and will be able to see a vision for your future that you hadn't imagined before.

Why be the type of person who waits and delays living your Big Life? Be the kind of person who takes the steps necessary to accomplish your goals and, over time, shows the world what consistent and focused effort can do for someone who starts small.

I'm not saying everything will be simple. In fact, the steps and activities I outline in these pages take hard work! But I can promise you that doing nothing will keep you right where you are, never progressing or moving forward toward the life you deserve.

The process of starting small that I share is time-tested and has worked over and over again for people of all ages. It is a process that, once you understand how it works, you can use repeatedly as you identify new goals and go after them. It will become a new way of looking at the world and attacking challenges. Your responses to obstacles will change as you start living in this new way.

You wouldn't have the desire for more in your head if you weren't meant to find a way to make it come true. In the pages ahead you'll find the foundation for creating a life you are happy with. I would encourage you to read the first three chapters in order. These lay the foundation for how to shift your thinking and create your plan of action. You'll understand the basics for the C.H.A.S.E. framework and how to apply it to your life. The remaining chapters cover different areas of your life, such as finances, career, and relationships. These chapters can be read in order or you can skip around to an area of your life that you want to get started on changing.

Chapters four through nine contain stories of people who have begun to live Big Lives and how to be creative as you think through plans of your own. The final chapter, "The Power of Stating Small" holds a challenge for you to start taking action today. You can find out more about the people in the stories as well as download any worksheets and challenge guides on my website, www.startsmalltolivebig.com

Let the Start Small framework guide you into living that Big Life you've been dreaming of.

I can't wait to hear about the Big Life you are about to create!

CHAPTER 1
CREATING YOUR VISION

The very best thing you can do for the whole world is to make the most of yourself. — Wallace D. Wattles

In 1983, Jim Valvano was the head coach at North Carolina State University. He had a vision to become the greatest basketball coach there ever was. When he was hired, he told the players that he had a dream to take them to the championship game. The team looked at him in disbelief. The Wolfpack had experienced loss after loss, and there was nothing obvious about how they played that would make anyone think he could get the job done and realize his dream.

But Coach V, as the team called him, believed in his vision and kept talking about it. Each year, he devoted an entire practice to celebrating just as they would when they won the championship. They didn't play any basketball that day. Coach V would pull out a ladder and have them practice cutting down the nets, just as they would do after winning the National Collegiate Athletic Association

(NCAA) tournament. Spending that much time, an entire practice with no basketball, was unheard of for a team in the Atlantic Coast Conference (ACC). But Coach V believed in the power of thoughts.

Three years into coaching the Wolfpack, the team made the ACC tournament, but with ten losses in their regular season it wasn't going to be easy to win. And if they wanted to make it to the NCAA tournament, that is what they needed to do. They won three straight games in that tournament, taking the title, and moving on to the NCAA tournament. This was it! This was what Coach V had been focused on his whole career. The Wolfpack went on to win six consecutive games at the NCAA tournament, four of which they won in the final minute. In that final game, Houston was favored to win, but the Wolfpack pulled through and the coach's vision was realized. After the game, with the crowd cheering, a ladder was rolled out and the team cut down the nets, just like they had in practice so many times before.

Know Where You Are Going

Having a vision is vital to knowing where you are going. It's hard to start if you have no idea what Living Big could really mean for your life. It's easy to say, "Well, I want a job I love, a happy marriage, and kids that are happy." But to define what that means for you is important. My version of a happy marriage may be different than yours, so defining *your* vision of a Big Life is vital for your path.

Several years ago I implemented a new morning routine, getting up before the rest of the house had awakened. It was great to have time just for myself. I spent the time reading, meditating, and visualizing my future. This helped me to start thinking bigger than I had been, and I found that spending time exposing myself to new ideas through books was really valuable.

But it wasn't until I decided to write down my dream life that things became clear for me. I realized I had been confusing what I wanted for myself with what I thought people expected me to want for myself. And I realized that when we understand what we want for our lives, instead of what we think would please others, we can truly start living a Big Life. So I decided to write every little detail about what a Big Life would include for me.

I took several hours and wrote down my perfect day. I wrote it as if I was a scriptwriter for a blockbuster movie, and every little detail would need to be provided so that it would come out exactly as I envisioned. What I thought would take ten minutes ended up taking close to three hours, but in the end, I had written out my dream day with such precision that I could see the shape of my home office window in my mind's eye, I could smell the ocean air, and I knew what direction I'd need to look to see the sunset. I knew who was in my home when I woke up and what type of friends stopped by. I knew my work, my plans, where I vacationed and even the types of photographs I had around my home.

My dream day, when it was all written out, wasn't what I expected. It was much different than the life I had been living but, more importantly, it was different than the life I had been telling myself I wanted to live.

Writing my dream day allowed me to envision my Big Life without fear of anyone else seeing it, judging me, or altering my view. What came out was so Me I felt like I'd just walked into a freezer — every part of my body was alive.

Every day for months, during those early morning hours I read my perfect day. Some days, I could see my vision so clearly and it felt so real, it brought tears to my eyes. The excitement and joy I felt for what was coming was undeniable.

I've talked with both happy, contented people living their Big Life and people who are looking for something more, and there is a distinct difference between the two. People living their Big Lives have a clear vision of what brings them happiness and what they want for their lives. People who are looking for more are just taking what comes in life without feeling in control of their direction.

Not knowing what our Big Life looks and feels like is one of the biggest ways we can shortchange ourselves. If I asked you what you wanted your life to look like in three or five years, you may have a vague idea. You may be clear in one or two areas, but I'm willing to bet other areas are left to chance. Maybe you are clear on what you want to do with your career or your relationship with your children but you have no idea what you want for your life with your partner, your adventure, or your health. You may have failed to dream about all areas of your life, focusing instead on just a few. You may even have ideas that aren't yours, but are what someone else would want for you — what you think you "should do."

Break the streak of spending your life being fuzzy on what you want your life to be. Get clear on your vision, find the authentic you, and be honest with what makes you jump for joy. Later, we'll work on developing the courage to act on the wishes of your soul but, for now, we have to learn to listen for them.

You may find that before you begin defining and living your Big Life, making some commitments can help you be authentic in deciding what you really want for yourself.

Be True to Yourself

It was New Year's Eve, a night when celebrations are everywhere and new hopes and dreams for the coming year are born. I had been planning this party for the past year and now the big day was here. We had decided to celebrate in Vermont, near my hometown; it was traditional for the bride to get married at home, after all.

The past few years had been full of change and there were moments I felt like I was on a carnival ride I wasn't sure how to slow down. Things spun in and out of focus as I worked on doing the small actions every day that I thought would bring me happiness.

Everyone from my soon-to-be husband's family came from New York. Friends arrived in packs and celebration mode was in full force. The night before, my fiancé partied with family friends, attending a big bachelor party. I stayed in with my sister and spent the night at the hotel getting our nails done and having dinner together. I was nervous, and my head was spinning. I knew I was supposed to feel over-the-moon excited. But I wasn't. I felt unsure of myself and uncomfortable.

It wasn't that Matt wasn't a great guy — he was. His family was great and he had good values. He had supportive parents, sisters, aunts and uncles, and role models to build an incredible life. I knew he would be a great dad, and I felt grateful to be accepted into a family again. I missed that — family. Looking back at that time now, I see that my spinning head, combined with my lack of stability and acceptance, caused me to ignore myself.

I ignored my own voice as I looked in the mirror and spoke out loud: "Betsy, if you get married, you're going to get divorced."

But the wheels were in motion, and so I stayed the course, not knowing where else I would land or what I would do.

I can see now that while I had been rushing from one thing to the next and trying to keep up with a schedule I had set for this event, I had begun to doubt myself. I talked badly about myself and ignored the inner voice that knows my truth. And I failed to grow.

A few years later, after a move to a new state and the purchase of a home, it was over. I'd fulfilled my prophecy of divorce and, at only 27, I knew I had a lot left to learn.

The years that followed were filled with internal conflict and a feeling of being unsettled. I knew that this leap hadn't been the right thing for me and that taking simple, small steps toward the kind of relationship I needed was where I should focus my attention. But the relationship I really needed was the relationship with myself. If I wanted to build meaningful relationships with others, I needed to better understand myself.

You may not have had a woman in a white dress staring back at you from a mirror, knowing you were doing everyone in your life a disservice, but maybe you've done something equally catastrophic. There are lots of ways we can fail ourselves. The important thing is to stop and find ways to move out of the habit of ignoring our inner voice. Then we can begin to be true to ourselves and develop our personal vision for a Big Life.

Be Kind to Yourself

My husband recently brought me to Myrtle Beach for a quick getaway. If you've never been to Myrtle Beach, think of any touristy beach with a boardwalk, restaurants, and gift shops. Condos, one after the other, line the main drag, and the beach is covered with big umbrellas and water activities for hire. It's a fun little beach and hyper busy during the tourist months.

One night, we wandered into a dueling piano bar and parked ourselves at a high-top table with a perfect view of what was about to go down. We were early, but soon the place was packed and the talent began getting ready to take the stage.

Two men, one looking to be in his 20's and the other in his 40's, were setting up. They had a system for how the night would run and they worked together to create a fun environment. It didn't take long before they were racking in tips with song requests and sending the crowd into a frenzy with their banter and friendly teasing of groups in the crowd.

Besides the music being fun, it was a sight to see from a business perspective. The two men worked the crowd, gave a great show, and got the whole room involved. But I kept noticing that, although clearly talented, most of the younger pianist's jokes were about himself. It was funny at first, as self-deprecating humor can be. But soon I started to feel sad.

We all do it — say things to ourselves we would never let anyone else say to us. Yet here he was, wickedly talented, clearly living in his zone of genius and having a great time, but still being mean to himself.

Now, in his defense, I'll point out that it was part of his shtick. But humor is never all about the joke. And I know we all do this same thing — thinking that negative self-talk will somehow motivate us to make changes or inspire us to become more.

It never works that way.

The brain is so powerful that it wants to create the experience you are telling it to expect. It wants to prove you right. Tell your brain that you're not very smart, and it will start showing you more situations where you don't seem very smart. Tell your brain that you have a unique perspective on things and it will shift to show you more of that unique perspective.

Focusing on what you *don't* want instead of what you *do* want can be a difficult habit to stop. When we look in the mirror, or get a low grade on an exam in school, or don't get chosen for a promotion at work, it can be difficult to see the positive and not focus on all the ways we think we have failed. How do we change and start focusing on our greatness? How do we cut the mean talk and start treating ourselves the way we would treat someone we love and respect?

Start by becoming aware of the negative words you use when you talk to yourself. Notice how you talk about yourself with others and when you talk to yourself during the day. Once you are aware, you'll start to notice things popping up throughout your day. Once you have awareness, catch yourself and shift your statement into something kinder. As you begin to notice where you are mean to yourself, create some regular "shifters" — positive words to replace the negative ones.

The trick to making this shift is that your words must be *believable*. Shifting your conscious thinking will also begin to shift your unconscious thinking.

I've always been athletic. When I was young, I played sports and spent lots of time outside being active. I also had big legs. Strong legs. The thigh-gap fashion trend was lost on me! My legs kept me from wearing skinny jeans, and I had to steer clear of certain fashion trends. I got into the habit of being down on myself about my legs. Every time I put on jeans I'd get annoyed. I'd complain in the mirror when I saw my thighs in shorts, and for a long time I used my big legs as just one more reason I wasn't "good enough" to have a Big Life.

I had to shift my thinking.

I had to learn to talk to myself in a positive but believable way. If every time I looked in the mirror I switched from saying, "My legs are big," to "My legs are thin," I wouldn't believe it, and my brain would simply disregard what I'd said (after it finished laughing!).

I needed to change my self-talk to *believable* self-talk. So I made the shift from, "My legs are so big!" to "Those are some strong legs! They are healthy and will take me all over the world when I'm ready." I'm no longer telling myself things that aren't true, I'm training myself to see the positive. Shifting my words helps me shift my focus to the positive, focusing on what I want instead of what I don't want.

Now I can be more focused on abundance and less on lack. When I make it a habit of doing this consciously, my brain will take over and start doing it unconsciously for me.

Making the small shift from "mean friend" to "kind friend" has had an incredible impact on how I live my life.

Now it's your turn. Here's how:

Begin by asking where in your life you are choosing hurtful words instead of helpful words. Watch your words for a few days and begin to make a list. I find it helpful to simply draw a line down the middle of a piece of paper to make two columns. In the left column, I write down the negative messages I notice I tell myself. When I have my list, I spend some time thinking about each of those negative messages and deciding how I can best shift them to the positive. I write the positive messages in the opposite column. Remember, just because I focused on the strength of my legs doesn't mean there isn't fat on them! That may be a fact, but I am shifting my focus to the positive. Make your list and shift each negative statement to a positive one.

When you are done, take a long, hard look at your list. Read through the positive list out loud. Soak the words into your mind, and realize that all the words on the positive side are *true*. Carry your list with you throughout the day. When you notice you are thinking something on the negative side, immediately shift to something from the positive side. At first, this may seem odd and may not come naturally. That's okay. If you remember it a minute later, practice shifting. Your brain will begin shifting on its own, just like you don't have to remind yourself to brush your teeth in the morning. You go into the bathroom in the morning and, as soon as you see the sink, you remember to brush. Brushing your teeth comes naturally and, soon, shifting to being kind to yourself will too.

Focus On Your Unique Strengths

My thumb has traveled a million miles on Instagram.

I follow people who post pictures of themselves in beautifully lit photos with perfectly combined outfits including just the right accessories. Their lives seem deliriously fabulous and color coordinated. I follow people who post inspirational quotes and messages that have amazing graphics created with years of Photoshop skills.

And lifters. I follow a lot of Olympic style lifters.

They do the Snatch and the Clean and Jerk. The lifting, the powerfulness of it, the strength and precision, when done right, is a thing of beauty. Their videos show training sessions with fit friends in the background cheering them on as they dive under the bar, which seems to sail effortlessly overhead, their abs glistening.

I didn't discover Olympic lifting until my late 30's, and now that I'm 45, I feel like I've come a long way.

I love my garage space. With the sun coming in at just the right angle, it's bright but not too hot. Even in the Atlanta summer sun, I feel happy and at peace. A few plates are scattered on the floor. There are no mats, or a fancy lifting platform, just the concrete covered in a dusting of hand chalk. I take my photos, too, with a tripod that was bent by a falling plate. All my videos are slightly crooked, and the weights I lift are much less than those in the videos. But I don't mind.

Lifting isn't just for my body; it's for my soul too.

I feel good about my lifting and what I am accomplishing in my little garage space. For me, lifting is spiritual. A chance to connect with myself. A time to think.

As my thumb scrolls a million miles, I find myself inspired, but there is something else.

The strange feeling of comparison. I may have just finished my own lifting session, and felt strong and happy, but when I start to scroll I suddenly feel as though I'm not enough.

Not strong enough. Not lean enough. Not successful enough. I started too late. I'm too old. I'm too quad dominate. (That's a thing!) Whereas I felt wonderful just a few short minutes before, now I feel "less than."

It's simple to feel good enough, when I'm in my garage and away from everyone while I work out every day — until I catch a glimpse of someone else and what they are lifting. *What they are becoming.*

And how could I not compare? How could I not scroll through the feed and see the amazing things that everyone else is doing and not feel that way? How do I see all the greatness out there, and not feel as if all the greatness is taken up? As if it's already been done, or someone is better, smarter, stronger — younger.

It doesn't matter if I'm talking about lifting, or posting on Instagram. We all have times when we compare ourselves to others.

I bet you do it too.

- With the other moms in the school pick-up line, who are always on time and involved with all their kids' projects and activities, while you are just trying to get to work before your boss notices you're late.
- With the man at work who comes up with the creative ideas you wish you'd thought of, leaving your old crappy ideas from last week feeling…well…crappy.
- With the other online business owners in your niche who have better websites, better logos, more clients, more… greatness.

So you go home and have a glass of wine and pretend you are just fine because, really, everyone around you is able to do it all so much better, why bother?

Because, the truth is, they *can't* do it all so much better. They can't do YOU in the specific and special way that YOU can do you.

There is something special about the way I post pictures with my tilted little camera on the bent tripod. Something different about the people I can inspire in my 45-year-old way. Something unique about the words I choose and the things I learn in my garage that I have to share.

There is something special about what *you* are doing every day too. It's normal to feel that sense of comparison or jealousy, but you don't have to let it define you.

There is no limit to greatness. It doesn't get "all used up" so there is nothing left for anyone else. There isn't a bucket with inspiration and gifts that gets drained by others finding their greatness before you do. There is no cap on supply. And even if there were, not everyone wants the same things from the bucket!

I may want to lift heavy weights, and you may want to play a great game of tennis. We all put our special spin on our slice of greatness, which makes it different than what anyone else is able to do.

It's special because it's YOU doing it.

Yes, those lifters may be farther along than I am in my quest for greatness but, instead of comparing myself, I remember they can't do it like I can. And I don't want to do it exactly like they do.

I use their progress to inspire me and drive me to be more like me. I appreciate their special gifts and I allow their videos to serve as inspiration for hard work and for doing things in my own way, instead of wanting to be someone else. I stop comparing.

That is how I'll find my greatness. And that's how you'll find yours too.

Focus on the special strengths only you can give to the world. Someone needs you to find your gifts and stay true to those gifts. *You* need you to drop the comparison, be aware of the stories you tell yourself, and allow others' progress to inspire you. You've got experiences and insight nobody else has. The way you see the world is unique, and just as you can learn from others' stories, someone needs to learn from yours.

Our feelings are a barometer to what's happening inside our mind. Because some feelings, like jealousy, are uncomfortable, we push them aside and choose to move our focus to something else. I'll encourage you to push through these feelings instead of going around them. Spend a minute when that feeling comes up and explore what that experience means for you.

I try hard to focus on gratitude in my life and, like many people, I say thanks before eating my evening meal. For some reason, doing this was making me emotional. I felt on the brink of tears some days, and it made me feel embarrassed and silly. So I decided to go through my emotion instead of around it. I stopped and felt my emotion and simply asked myself, "Why?" I answered that I was grateful for the food. Why? Because many people don't get healthy food. Why? Because I appreciated where the food came from. Why? Because I know how hard farming is, and I appreciate the work that went into giving me this meal. Why? Because my father grew up as a farmer, and when I say grace for the food I think of the farmers and then of him and, since I don't see him very much, it makes me miss him.

Being grateful for my food made me miss my dad, and I never would have recognized this as the source of my emotion before asking myself the questions. Now that I have the knowledge, I can do something about it. I can reach out and call my dad. I can plan more visits to see him, and I can share with him what I'm feeling, maybe bringing us closer together.

Listen to your feelings, don't push them aside. Ask yourself "why" and see what comes up for you.

Having a clear vision for your life will make the journey simpler. Decisions on what road to take will be easier if you know where you're headed. Staying the course through life's bumps in the road will seem more stable when you are being true to yourself, when you can be kind to yourself on the journey and can learn to focus and appreciate your unique strengths. Establishing these habits will build a solid foundation for you to begin creating your Big Life.

CHAPTER 2

KNOW WHAT YOU BELIEVE

You attract the right things when you have a sense of who you are. — Amy Poehler

It was just after New Year's Day. Avoiding the rush at the local franchise gym, I wandered into a freshly opened CrossFit Box (CrossFit calls their gyms "boxes"), not far from my house. I'd heard a few people talking about CrossFit and was curious what it was all about. It hadn't become mainstream yet and the word on the street was that this type of workout was so strenuous it would send you headfirst into the trash can, vomiting your dinner — if you did it right. If you aren't familiar with CrossFit, it's a fitness craze in which people push themselves to their limits with hard workouts.

Even though it sounded brutal, I had always been up for an athletic challenge, and the fact that nobody else was really doing it yet made it appeal to me even more. Being a single mom, I wasn't able to work out whenever I wanted. I missed having that freedom, but when I walked into the Box, I noticed they had a small waiting area up front. Olive had just turned seven, and she was into art and loved to read. I knew she would be able to sit still if I decided to try it out.

It was quiet. *Anyone here?* I wondered. The door had been propped open so I gave a quick scan of the room.

"Hello?" I called out.

As I came around the desk, I saw a man in his 20's with a dirty mop of blond hair. I assumed he was the manager. Fast and furious, he threw himself down into a push up and then jumped up explosively, clapping his hands overhead. He was red-faced and looked exhausted.

"Almost done…just one minute!" he called out to me so I'd know he saw me. I waited patiently.

He was down on the ground again, jumping up and clapping overhead, but this time, it registered: what I was seeing was truly unique. My eyes focused on the clap. Jumping up again, his arms pounded together, but where hands should have been were just two stubs. His arms, muscular and defined, ended right at his elbow. He threw himself down on the floor again. Nothing below his knee, I noticed now, and understood more about the name of the gym I had just walked into: *No Excuses.*

The man finished his workout in a heap on the floor. Sweating profusely, he dragged himself over to shake my hand and introduce me to his gym.

"I'm Kyle." He offered me his stub. Under any other circumstances I may not have known what to do, but Kyle was so at ease, it wouldn't have mattered if I shook his stub or gave him a high five. I grabbed his arm and we instantly became friends.

"Ready to try it out? he asked.

Kyle was born with congenital amputation. Simply put, it means he has shortened limbs. It's all he has known and, as I got to know him, I realized just now normally he lives his life.

Kyle has created ways to do just about everything that people with hands and feet can do. He can also do things many people with hands and feet *can't* do. He has a drive and focus that many people lack, and an uncompromising belief system that supports his dreams and goals. Kyle lives Big.

He once explained to me that he thinks people are made by the adversity they face in their lives. That we each have a challenge to overcome in our lifetimes. The key is to be fearless. Challenges are what builds our character and defines who we are.

So how did Kyle come to the realization that his birth defect was really a blessing? How did he start out being different from all his friends, being picked on by some, and instead of getting bitter, building a life in which he inspires others, owns a fitness center, and speaks all over the world encouraging others to drop their excuses? It all comes down to his beliefs and how he works with them.

Growing up, Kyle's parents saw the potential he had for his life. They wanted his life to be just as full and independent as *any* of his friends, and so they treated Kyle just like any other kid. They required he learn basic skills that may have been difficult to learn at first. Soon Kyle was proficient at simple things most of us take for granted; using silverware, cooking, and taking part in everyday activities just like other kids became simple over time. When he wanted to play sports, his parents didn't discourage him or hold him back, but instead pushed him forward. They didn't allow the opinions of outsiders to infect their hopes for their son to live a full and meaningful life.

The message Kyle heard, from early on, is that there are no excuses. He not only had the ability, he had the requirement to learn to be independent.

Were there times Kyle felt like he couldn't do everything his parents asked of him? Of course. But their belief made him push through, and his success reinforced the truth of their ideas and made his belief in himself grow.

We all struggle to believe in ourselves at times. We think we can't do something, or we think a Big Life isn't for us. Different areas of our lives may be more challenging than others. For some of us, our struggle shows itself mainly in our relationships or our health or in our careers. For all of us, lack of belief keeps us from living the Big Life we deserve.

I remember, as a kid, hearing the story about how circus elephant trainers were able to train those big giant elephants to stay put in the barn. The trainers would take the elephants as infants and tie them with big huge ropes to the barn. When the elephants tried to pull away, they struggled and eventually gave up. Later, the trainers didn't even need large ropes to contain them. The elephants believed they couldn't break free, so they stopped trying.

Our belief systems can push us forward, like Kyle's did, or hold us back like the baby elephants. Our experiences and influences are what create our beliefs. The key to moving forward is finding out what beliefs are truly holding you back and where those beliefs come from. Awareness is the first step to changing your life.

Awareness is the Answer

There is good news! You can not only become aware of how you think, you can begin to understand how your thinking holds you back. You don't have to go to years of therapy to undo what's firmly in your head. Instead, you need to listen to your internal conversation and ask yourself questions. This journey of awareness can be eye-opening and bring you joy as you begin to unpack beliefs that no longer benefit you.

Because limiting beliefs are so destructive, but so simple to change, everyone would progress if they understood how they truly viewed the world. To support you in accomplishing this, I'm going to share some simple tools that will help you stop, listen, and assess.

After you become more aware, you will find it easier to identify what you want to change and how to start shifting your thinking. This isn't a one-time shot of awareness, identification, and shifting.

This is an ongoing process, because beliefs are continuously being formed. As you practice, it will become easier and easier to identify limiting beliefs, and beliefs that you didn't even know you held will make their way to the surface.

Understanding the Different Kinds of Beliefs

Now you know that beliefs can hold you back or help you, but you may not understand WHAT a belief is. This is both an easy and complex question. When it comes down to it, beliefs are everything you think you know about every single part of the world.

Here's an example. Perhaps you are looking at your life right now and thinking, *I have issues with my finances.* In order to change the issues you have with your finances and make progress, you must first understand what you really believe about your finances. This is where beliefs can get kind of tricky because we've fooled ourselves into thinking, *Well I'm just not good at budgeting,* or, *I am bad at saving.* But not being good with money or being bad at saving is not what's really holding you back. What's holding you back are your underlying *beliefs* about money — what you think about money itself.

You experience your reality based on all the things that have happened to you in your life and, in turn, your reality defines how you experience the world. If you aren't aware of why you think the way you do, if you have no idea that your past is filtering your vision of today, and if you have beliefs you aren't even aware of, how can you be in control of your own life? Instead, every day you are just reacting to patterns you learned a long time ago and that may not even be benefiting you anymore. You can only be free when you know what you really believe.

When you start digging, many beliefs will be obvious to you, and some will be more covert. To simplify, let's look at the four belief definitions below. Then we'll talk about taking the steps to change them.

1. The Obvious. These are the beliefs you are already aware of. Someone asks you what you think about dogs, and you already know. It's on the tip of your tongue. You think dogs are great companions and you love them. Or maybe you are afraid of dogs, but as soon as someone asks you what you think, you *know*. No doubts. This belief is obvious to you. Keep in mind that just because a belief is obvious doesn't mean it's serving you; it just means it's easy to identify and connect with how you feel about that topic. You can get to the root of it easily.

2. The Sneaky. This belief is one that sneaks out when you aren't expecting it. And when it slips out in conversation, you recognize it, but it doesn't seem like something you would say.

The Sneaky may reveal itself in something as innocent as talking to a friend who is going on vacation, and you find yourself saying, "Wow, must be nice." Look deeper at the power behind those words. "Must be nice" leads to "but I wouldn't know, because vacations take money I don't have," which is actually expressing an underlying belief about money.

Or perhaps, "but I wouldn't know because I can never get time away," which would be an underlying belief about time and your lifestyle limitations.

The Sneaky can be fun to catch, because it's unconscious and gives you a real glimpse into deep-seated beliefs that you may not have realized you had.

3. The Hand-Me-Down. This belief is something you got from your past. It may be from your parents or another family member or even a close family friend that you spent a lot of time with growing up. The Hand-Me-Down can be self-limiting, because it's generally not something you decided to believe about life. It's just a belief that you mindlessly adopted as truth while you were busy learning about the world.

The Hand-Me-Down reveals itself when someone asks you why you said or did something a certain way and you think, *because that's how we always did things*, or, *because that's what my dad told me*.

4. The Baby. The baby is a belief you have adopted recently. Even as adults we are taking information, making assessments, and determining what is "truth" for us. Our brains are constantly making assessments about our surroundings and environment and new beliefs are a normal byproduct of those judgments. The Baby can be a belief you adopted by breaking down an older, limiting belief and replacing it with the new baby. Or it could be a belief you adopted after having an experience that had a deep impact on you.

Beliefs come into our lives for many different reasons and in many different ways. The goal is to become aware of and understand what you believe and why you believe it. Learning to be aware will help you strengthen beliefs that support you and quickly identify and change the ones that don't. It will become easier to find your motivation and work toward the shifts you want to see in your life. In Kyle's life, his parents worked to instill beliefs that he could do or be anything he wanted in his life. But what if you are an adult and on a path that isn't serving you? What if you want to change but don't know how to get to the bottom of it?

What DO You Believe?

To gain a better understanding of your beliefs, select an area of your life that you want to work on and ask yourself five questions:
- What do I think about that topic?
- What do I think about myself in relation to that topic?
- What do I think about the rest of the world in relation to that topic?
- Where did these beliefs come from?
- Do these beliefs empower or limit me?

For example, if you struggle with your finances, ask yourself,
1. What do I think about finances? You may respond, "Money doesn't grow on trees."
2. What do I believe about myself in relation to finances? "I just can't stick to a budget." Or, "I will never have lots of money."

3. What do I believe about the world in relation to money? You might answer something like, "People who have money are greedy and don't care about others."
4. Where did these beliefs come from? "My dad always said we never have enough."
5. Do these beliefs empower or limit me? If you like money, and you wish you had more, these beliefs are not empowering but are limiting your goals and how you'd like to see your life.

Once you get those beliefs out in the open and are gaining clarity, you may begin to feel emotions you didn't expect to feel. Anger or frustration may make you nervous. This is the point at which you start to change those old patterns and find ways to punch holes in those beliefs.

For example, take the belief that "People who have money are greedy and don't care about others." You can easily do a Google search and find people who have made lots of money, who have non-profits and share their money with every kind of charitable cause.

What if you believe you don't have money because you didn't go to college? You can find many successful people who didn't attend or graduate from college. From designer Ralph Lauren to Bill Gates, Simon Cowell, and Coco Channel to Richard Branson, some of the richest people in the world, didn't finish college. They are no better than you are. (If you don't believe that statement, get to work breaking down the that limiting belief!)

You might also think of a time when you did make money. When was that? Were you greedy? Did you not care about people?

Once you understand how beliefs work, you will begin to notice when old patterns show up, and you will be able to stop them. For example, noticing when you are overeating to calm down feelings of not having control over your life allows you to make a conscious choice about why you are eating and if you want to continue or make a shift. Noticing when you are working all weekend in order to avoid having a confrontation, because you believe confrontations are bad, allows you to stop that behavior and make a decision about how you want your life to be. Being aware allows you to determine your behavior instead of acting unconsciously while thinking you are in control. Awareness allows you to develop beliefs that empower you to live the Big Life you want.

Tidying Up

As you begin to identify your limiting beliefs and punch holes in them, keep in mind that our brains don't understand the differences between physical danger and emotional turmoil. As you start exploring your beliefs and questioning yourself, it will seem uncomfortable. It's counterintuitive to our brains to think through belief systems that have been working. According to our brains, "working" means keeping us alive and safe, so your brain will start to reject this new thinking, and your amygdala may start to kick in.

As I mentioned before, the amygdala is critical to the process of survival. It controls our "fight or flight" response, alerting us to danger when we need to be ready to protect ourselves. When it's set off, like an alarm in your head, all other processes shut down temporarily to allow all your energy and focus to go into one thing and one thing only — staying alive. Your ability to be creative, rationalize, and make educated decisions with your mind are shut off completely. Your brain takes over and is fully involved in helping you escape from danger.

This response comes in pretty handy when there is an accident or we need all our resources to make life altering decisions quickly. But, for everyday living, the amygdala can screw with our goals and set us up for failure. Any time we get uncomfortable, striving for something new, or our regular patterns are changed, the amygdala leaps into action.

When this happens, even though we have the best intentions, it's hard to fight with nature. Processes like rational thinking and creative troubleshooting, processes we need when faced with a challenge to our goals, are shut down to give more energy to being alert and ready for action.

We may think we are ready to challenge our belief systems, but then our brains freeze. We get overwhelmed with change and taking that action turns seems overwhelming. We can't find ways to make the change work and so we slip back into our comfortable old habits and ways of thinking, which makes our amygdala very happy and able to rest. That's when the rest of our brain starts to function again, and we beat ourselves up because we weren't able to follow through.

Starting small is a trick to beat the amygdala. It's a way to tiptoe past the sleeping giant and make a move toward our goals. When we do just a little bit, so little it would be silly not to follow through (helping to create a new habit), but not so big that it makes any sort of waves at all, we can start to change without tripping the wire for our flight-or-flight response.

Something as small as just putting on workout clothes every day, instead of diving into a full cardio workout plan, can allow your threshold to change so that moving closer and closer to your goal isn't cause for alarm. No red flags are raised doing it this way and, as your brain gets used to this activity, you simply add on a little more. When the alert threshold is changed, your motivation is changed and getting going doesn't seem so hard, because your brain is starting to work with you instead of against you.

You can apply this to any area of your life.

Remember: start small, do just a little bit, and allow the threshold of what you can handle expand in a natural way.

When I was beginning the process of identifying my beliefs I experienced a lot of turmoil. I found I was really edgy. I got frustrated easily and was short with my husband. I was angry that I had lived my life for so long, not understanding how I felt about things. I felt like I had been a zombie, thinking I had freedom of choice when really that wasn't the case.

I learned that although I tended to focus on the positive in my life, for me it was also a coping mechanism to ignore the beliefs that had repeatedly held me back. Imagine the energy it must have taken to keep myself in the dark for so long! When I decided I was no longer willing to live like that, I acted against what my gut said to do. My brain and all my physiology told me to just ignore the work. Go back to how I was. I was fine!

But I knew that wasn't the case.

A few small steps I took helped me get over this reaction. One was to remind myself that I was safe. I told myself this whenever I felt that nervous energy come up as I did the work. I would say it out loud so I could hear myself, and sometimes I would imagine my mother saying it to me in the voice she used to comfort me when I was a little girl.

I also reminded myself that I didn't want to live the way I was. I wanted to change. This reminder allowed my guard to go down long enough for me to get inside my mind and start sifting through the useless junk.

Last year, after I read *The Magic of Tidying Up* by Marie Kondo, I cleaned out my whole house. Room after room, I emptied junk drawers and cleaned out closets, reorganizing in a way that made sense and bringing order to the house. Everything works now, and the way I reorganized fostered continued order. It was a system that changed my outer life. Working on becoming aware of and changing what we believe reorganizes our inner lives.

Shine the Light

This year when school started for my daughter Olive, we were adjusting to a new schedule. The bus came early in the morning and, to be sure everyone was ready for our day, I would get up at 5:00 a.m. This was about 45 minutes earlier than I usually got up. When I came downstairs that first morning, I noticed a swarm of ants by my back door in the kitchen. I opened the back door and shooed them out, hoping that would take care of the problem until I could get the exterminators to come.

If I hadn't gotten up so early, I never would have seen the ants. It was as though they knew when I usually turned on the lights and had been gathering by my back door for weeks without me noticing. I imagined they all chatted and checked the clock, running to their hiding place before they could be detected each morning. But once the light shone on them, and I saw them, they couldn't hide. I was aware and now had the ability to make my house a cleaner, ant-free environment.

It's just that way in our brains too. We may not realize the swarm of thoughts and beliefs holding us back and clouding our vision. But once we are alerted, and the light shines on them, we can get to work and start making the small shifts necessary to move toward our Big Lives.

CHAPTER 3

C.H.A.S.E. YOUR BIG LIFE

Rene Godefroy spent the first seven years of his life in a tiny village in Haiti. Born into extreme poverty, his life was hard. He grew up without what we would consider necessities: running water, electricity and plumbing. When Rene was only nine months' old, his mother left him with a neighbor so she could go to Port-au-Prince to find work, hoping to bring Rene with her in a short amount of time and provide him a better life.

Living with a neighbor in a tiny hut, Rene's childhood memories are mainly of misery, illness and pain. His little body was so riddled with sickness many of the villagers didn't believe he would live to be an adult. He didn't have any medical care, and he was routinely teased and ridiculed, surviving by eating mainly breadfruit he found in the village.

When he was seven, his mother finally called for him to join her in the city. Although she was doing the best she could to try to build them a better life, their home was a small shack infested with rats and cockroaches. He begged on the street for money, and they struggled to survive.

While out begging one day, he met some tourists who patted him on the head and gave him a dime. In that brief interaction, something incredible happened in Rene's life — he began to dream. He started to think about what life might be like outside of Haiti. He started to wonder about the world that other people came from, and he hoped there was something out there for him too.

By the time Rene had turned 21, that dream was becoming a reality. Not only was Rene starting small, he was starting with close to nothing. He came to America, with only $5 and a small suitcase with two shirts and a pair of pants. Landing in Miami Florida, Rene spent his money on a bucket and some soap and started asking if he could wash cars on the street.

Rene would wash cars outside the bank building and look up and think, *Someday I'm going to make it to the top of that building.* Right then, he may have been washing cars, but he knew he hadn't come all this way to have his story end there. Working away, day by day, he trusted in a better future.

Rene knew he had to learn English to advance in the United States, so he obtained some children's picture books. He committed to learning three words from the books every day. Banana, apple, whatever words were shown in his books, he would write on his hands and begin to repeat.

He worked hard until he was able to get a better job, moving forward from job to job, always learning more and committing to taking small steps toward his goals. Eventually he got a job working as a bellman for a large hotel. As the guests came in, he would notice what they were reading and jot down the names of the books. Then he would find and read each book as fast as he could.

Eventually, Rene knew that his calling was to inspire others, to show them that their past didn't have to equal their future, and that doing your best at the work you are doing today is the true highway to success. Today, Rene has gone from living in Haiti, riddled with illness and discomfort, to living a life full of purpose and clarity. Rene travels all over the country to share his story and to give people hope that no unpleasant condition is permanent.

I first met Rene and heard his message a decade ago, when he stood on the stage in front of me at an event in California. His message stuck with me ever since, as I learned that we all have the ability to overcome our past and do great things. My past didn't equal my future — if I started making changes now.

You have that ability too, to get from where you are to where you want to go. Even for Rene, change didn't happen overnight. It happened in tiny, incremental steps, each one building on the next. There were times he wasn't sure what his path was, but he just kept trying new things, learning and taking leaps of bravery. Each step showed him the way to the next, and soon his purpose was discovered. Were there setbacks and disappointments? Absolutely. But the persistent focus on where he was going and a belief that he could get there is what makes his story different from those of other kids in his small village.

There have probably been times when you have had a clear vision for a better life, but you also had doubt. Maybe you knew what you wanted in a relationship or in your career, but you just never felt like you were getting anywhere. The feeling of "spinning your wheels" can be a difficult one to overcome. Those tend to be the times when we just give up. We throw in the towel and decide this life we've dreamt up just isn't for us. Maybe other people get to have Big Lives, but that won't happen for us. We think it's just time to move on.

Rene and I went to lunch recently and he told me a story about a young woman he met on a visit back to Haiti. She came to him and told him that a friend of hers had recently taken her own life, and the young woman told Rene, "If she had seen you speak just a few months ago, this never would have happened." Rene wasn't sure what to say, but she continued, "Do you know why I tell you that? It is because I was on the same path, but now that I have heard you I have hope for what my life can be."

Imagine if Rene had given up. Imagine if the times he felt like he was getting nowhere, and felt like he was spinning his wheels, he had simply given up. Nobody would have faulted him. Overcoming all that he experienced in his small village in Haiti must have been overwhelming, but he found the strength to keep pushing forward.

Rene had the ability to impact someone in a great way and so do you. Maybe it's not a stranger, maybe it's someone close to you. Things may be difficult, but the tide will change. As Rene would say, "No condition is permanent."

Too Big

You may already have a vision for what Living Big is to you. And maybe you feel overwhelmed by how much needs to change in your life to get where you want to be. You may feel like the chasm is too wide to cross and feel defeated before you even begin.

The problem with thinking big is that we are *looking* too far ahead. Keep dreaming big, that's the good part. But *looking* too far forward can be overwhelming. Instead of focusing on how far you need to travel, focusing on the small steps you can take now will help the distance become manageable.

This is where you can use the C.H.A.S.E. framework to push toward what you want.

C.H.A.S.E. Create. Help. Attain. Start. Examine.

I am about to share with you my proven framework for defining your Big Life and creating the small steps you can take to begin living it. For the following exercises, pull out (or copy) the C.H.A.S.E. worksheet from the "Worksheets and Resources" section in the back of the book. You can also download the worksheet from www.StartSmallToLiveBig.com

Start Small, Live Big

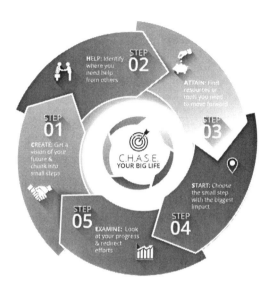

The C.H.A.S.E. Framework

Create

The Create step is the first in the C.H.A.S.E. framework and one of the most important. This is the beginning of being aware of where you are and of where you want to go. It's such a vital step, yet one many people bypass. When you skip this step all kinds of bumps in the road show up that could have been avoided. Taking the time to sit down and Create is important for your success.

The process will be the same for each area in your life, but we are going to focus on each one individually, so that you are clear on what needs to happen to move the needle forward in that particular area. Start by choosing the area that would have the biggest impact on your life right now. It could be health, relationships, or parenting. Maybe you want to work through a specific relationship with your parents or your husband, focus on your career or on finances. Whatever you choose, the Create process is where to begin.

At the top of the C.H.A.S.E. worksheet write a detailed description of what you want to change and the obstacles you think may be holding you back. Writing out your description of where you are will help you become clear on where you are right now and you may notice some things that are working for you already.

At the bottom of the page describe your vision of Living Big in this area, leaving room in the body of the page to brainstorm small steps. Living Big doesn't have to be a great adventure of change; it can involve a small change that would have a big impact on your happiness. Perhaps Living Big is simply having dinner with your family or increasing communication with your spouse. It could be to have a small savings account set up or sticking to your budget.

Everybody's Big Life is different. And your Big Life vision will be different now than it will be a year from now or five years from now. Creating a vision for your future is important — otherwise you are running through your days not knowing what you intend for your life or what would make you happy and fulfilled.

After you have written down your Big Life vision, you can begin brainstorming. This is the fun part, where you allow yourself to dream about what you *can* do.

Start by setting a timer for ten minutes and then brainstorm, writing down all the small steps you could take that will bring you from where you are at the top of the page, to your Big Life at the bottom of the page. Don't stop until the timer goes off! I love using a timer because it allows my mind to keep searching. You have all sorts of great ideas, but if you only write down what is on the top of your mind, you'll never dig down and find the good stuff. Only the ideas you've probably already thought of will emerge, and the great ideas, deep in your subconscious, will stay where they are.

Of course, taking action is where the magic happens, but don't let that slow you down in this step. Just because you write an action down doesn't mean you have to do it, so be free and creative and write down even the wild and wacky ideas. You can decide later what actions you think will really help you.

When I am having trouble identifying the steps I need to take, I find it helpful to look at the situation from another perspective, taking myself out of the equation and putting myself as the helper instead. I think, *If someone came to me with a similar issue, what would I think the steps should be?* I think through what sort of advice or information I would share and it helps me break through a trouble spot during my Create phase.

Help

Now that your list is complete, look it over and see what stands out as something you wouldn't be able to do alone. It's okay to get help when you need it. Maybe you would need to get professional help in a certain area, or you simply need someone to watch your kids so you can complete a step. Maybe asking a friend for help by getting feedback would help to move forward.

Circle any item on your list that you would need to reach out and get help with in order to accomplish. This small action of acknowledging that you don't have to do everything alone will calm your brain.

My friend Stephanie was developing her list and realized that it was time she looked for a new job. She had been working at her job for over four years and felt like she'd made a substantial impact, but also knew there was a "next step" for her career that she wasn't going to find with her current employer. Doing this exercise made her realize that she was going to have to take a leap to get out of her rut and begin feeling like she was living up to her full potential. When she made her list, including all the small steps she could think of, she realized that she was going to need help searching for a job. Reaching out to a recruiter would help her achieve this goal faster than doing it on her own. When she came to this realization, it freed her from the stagnation she had felt before, and she knew someone else was working on her behalf. Just a simple shift in realizing where she could get help made her feel like her Big Life was in reach.

Attain

When you started this brainstorming process you were bound to come up with actions that would help you move in the direction you want to go, but you don't have the knowledge or resources to start. What do you need to Attain to move forward? Do you need to research for more information, obtain resources, or learn more? Underline the ideas on your list that will require you to Attain something in order to accomplish them.

One of my girlfriends was interested in creating an online course to share her knowledge in career advancement. She had worked hard to create a following and was sharing ideas every day that helped people move from dead-end jobs to careers they loved.

She started the process of creating her course, but couldn't get the video right. She was always looking off to the side, couldn't remember her lines, or just felt like it looked choppy and out of sorts. She asked others who created courses how they did it and found she needed to attain a teleprompter. She took their suggestions, found one online, and now has an incredible course to share that is professional and easy to watch. If she hadn't taken time to map out her plan and learn what was missing, she never would have found the missing piece to make it a success.

Taking the steps you need to move forward may involve attaining resources. Once you have this realization, your mind will start to notice and find ways to help you attain what you need.

Start

There is no better time than right now! This step is where you take action. Review your list, including all the items you have circled and underlined, and decide where to get started. Draw a box around two or three steps that would have the biggest impact on your life right now. If a step feels risky, that just means the task isn't small enough. Is there a way to break that idea into smaller bits that would be so simple it would be silly not to do them? For example, if your idea is to reorganize your kitchen, can you do one drawer a day? If you want to run a 5k, can you start by walking to the end of the driveway? If you want to keep your car clean, can you start by working on keeping just the cup holders in order? Think about what you can do that would have an impact on your life but take under 10 minutes. Make the actions ridiculously easy so you have no reason you can't take consistent, daily steps toward your goal.

Now, add your selected steps to your calendar this week. If you only have time to do one task, that's okay! Doing one small step each day will move you forward toward that Big Life vision you have in mind.

My mother-in-law came over one Christmas a few years ago and brought with her every comic book and toy that my husband had in his entire childhood. Her car was packed and she was ready to move it all out of her house. They say your kids aren't ever really out of your house until their belongings are out of the basement, and now that he was 40, she was ready! We unpacked and moved everything to Craig's office in the basement. It was totally overwhelming, and I think Craig avoided the basement for a few months, but finally we decided living a Big Life meant being in control of our stuff.

He decided that he would put away or throw out one thing from one box every day. He didn't have to complete five boxes a day, or even one whole box, just one item. It took less than five minutes and, over time, the boxes started to disappear. Clutter was no longer taking over his office and he felt in control.

Examine

As you continue your process toward the Big Life, periodically examine your progress. Setting up a goal and not touching base with where you are for six months or a year allows too much time for you to go off the rails. Setting up regular "check-ins" with someone that can hold you accountable or with yourself is a smart way to be sure you are staying on track and not straying too far from the plan.

I had a friend in high school who decided to become an airline pilot. He went to flight school and worked toward his dream and now flies for a major airline, crisscrossing all over the United States. If he were flying from Los Angeles to visit me in Atlanta, but the nose of his airplane was 1% off course, by the time he got to the east coast he would be on track to land in South Carolina. Just 1% would set him off target 92 feet for every mile he traveled. If he were off track, it would be much easier to periodically adjust and land in the right place than to go all way to Charleston and then realize his mistake. Check-ins for our lives work the same way — they prevent you from making errors in your flight path that will take you to a destination you don't want.

I like Sunday night check-ins. This allows me to plan my week, add in my "start activities," and chat with my family about how I can help them and what they can do for me to make it a great week. I recommend you schedule time weekly to check in with yourself and your family and layout your plan for the week ahead.

If during your check-in you find you have gotten off your intended path, that's okay. Reexamining and changing your plan isn't failure, it's progress. Movement forward. That's why we stop at regular intervals to examine where we are to be sure we get back on track before we've strayed too far.

Avoiding Distractions

At my house, we have two dogs and a cat. One dog, Miley, is old and sweet. She'll stay in bed until noon if you let her, and she just wants to sit with you cuddle. She's only 14 pounds and she fits right on the couch or under your chair with no problems at all.

Henry, on the other hand, is about six months' old. He's fun and vivacious! He loves you so much, he wants to talk to you and play and, if you are home, he just wants to be with you! He's about

55 pounds and sometimes he drinks water just to drip it all over the floor and then play in it.

I struggle with the chaos of Henry at times. I love animals but found that I prefer animals that are old enough to be independent. I love that Miley is ready for love when I'm done working but Henry seems like a toddler I need to take care of all day. But how on earth do I get peace now? How do I get to where I want to be from where I am now?

It sounds silly, but this has been an overwhelming problem for me while writing this book. I struggled to balance the different needs of everyone (human and non-human) in the house while still accomplishing the goals I had set for myself.

So I did the C.H.A.S.E. exercise for myself. I set the timer. At the top of my list I wrote where I was: "chaos with the animals." At the bottom I wrote "peace and harmony." In between, I brainstormed ideas. Some of these ideas were crazy and some were great, but I just let my mind go to see what I could come up with.

When the timer went off I had a variety of ideas ranging from "that could work" to "am I insane?" I thought about putting him in his crate a few hours a day, working at a coffee shop, sitting on the front steps to get away, wearing earplugs, and bringing him for a walk before I write. Wearing Henry out, I finally decided, would help have the biggest impact. I decided to run him outside every morning. I'm not a super runner, but I've wanted to get my cardio exercise so I decided I'd start by walking him (not running since that would be a leap) an extra ten minutes every day.

That seems like such a small thing, but ten minutes a day, adds up to over an hour a week. That's close to five hours a month of extra walking for Henry. I reasoned that would help his energy level, as well as help him connect with me and learn to listen, if I also worked with him on the leash. The cardiovascular activity would help me too. It could even help with my stress levels. Only ten minutes a day (who doesn't have 10 minutes?) would add 60 HOURS a year to my exercise time. Such a big impact for such a small change. In addition,

I could use the time to listen to music to improve my mindset, podcasts to help me learn, or just be quiet in meditation as I walked.

I started in and, within just a few weeks, we increased from going to the end of my street, to the edge of my neighborhood, to the next neighborhood over every morning. Within a month, I was alternating walking and running between houses and feeling less stressed than ever. Now walking him first thing in the morning is one of the favorite parts of my day, and sometimes I do it after dinner too! If I had started out running him, I never would have lasted more than a day or two, but now I have a new habit and have managed to meet more of my neighbors in the process.

At the end of my first month, I realized I had walked Henry 34 miles using this simple process. I was surprised, because it felt so effortless, and it had a big impact on his energy level. He was calmer, started listening to direction, and I am now motivated to keep the walking schedule because I see the payoff with his happiness.

It's The Little Things

Completing the C.H.A.S.E. exercise has helped me over and over again. How many small action steps can you put in the space between where you are right now and your Big Life? It's those small steps that take you in the right direction. You can use a new C.H.A.S.E. worksheet for each area of your life, deciding what you need to focus on to build toward what you want. It may be that, initially, you pick one area to work on, but, over time, you'll see you can manage working on two or three areas at a time. You may have areas that overlap, and working on one area gives you results in two.

Give yourself a chance to grow and understand what a Big Life really means to you. Take the time to start with developing your Big Life vision as we discussed in chapter one. From there, you can break down the parts and start to focus on where you'll have the most impact. A Big Life is different for each of us, but you will never get there if you don't know where you are going. Be flexible and know that as you reach milestones your definition of your Big Life may change. There is no right or wrong. Your Big Life will be different from mine, but nobody else can do things just the way you can.

Once you are clear on your destination, become the person who lives that Big Life. Focus on the positives that will take you where you want to go. Give yourself time to work toward that life and don't get sidetracked when things get difficult. Instead, stop and break actions down into small steps you can take each day. That Big Life is waiting for you. Even if you are busy or overwhelmed with where you are right now, be true to yourself by finding small ways to work toward the greater life in store for you.

CHAPTER 4
AT ALL COSTS

There isn't a "one size fits all" when it comes to making decisions for our lives. Each of us wants something different, and our paths to achieve those goals will vary too. The area of finances is no exception. You may want to focus on this area of your life and decide what you want the outcomes to be. As I talked with people who were doing creative things to start small in their lives, I found how they made decisions about money to be very personal and unique. In this chapter, I share a few stories of people I found who are Living Big in unique ways when it comes to finances, proving that there is no one way to C.HA.S.E. your Big Life.

Outside the Neighborhood

Heather had her first child when she was 22. Eight years and four kids later, she and her husband Graham found themselves in a situation different from any they ever could have imagined.

I met up with them to hear more about their story at a recreational vehicle (RV) park just outside of Atlanta. Graham was renovating an RV a few doors down from where Heather and the kids were spending their morning, cleaning house and getting ready for the weekend. Like so many young couples, Graham and Heather want their kids to have great experiences growing up. They want their children to have an appreciation for nature and understand the importance of family. They want to teach them to search for what will bring them happiness and to find their passions.

Several years ago, Graham and Heather opened a CrossFit gym. They wanted to make an impact on peoples' lives and feel like they were doing something that mattered. Graham loved the coaching. He was able teach his clients skills that helped them become more fit, as well as to create better body-movement habits they could take with them into old age. Together, Graham and Heather created a community with its own unique personality. People who came into their gym felt the difference and were inspired to be open and learn from them both.

But having a small business had its challenges, and Heather and Graham struggled to find balance with the ups and downs of starting a gym from scratch. Some months were great, and they felt they were on a roll. But in other stretches business was painfully slow, and the financial stress was taking its toll. Graham described to me his thoughts on this stress and how it was so much different than other kinds of stress: "I found it easier to deal with some stressors in my life, like the stress from kids or jobs I had in the past. I found those stressors went to bed when I went to bed, but financial stress — that kept me up at night."

Throughout the few years their business was open, Heather and Graham struggled to keep money in the business and provide for their family, eventually losing their home. It was a tough reality, but they decided to focus on what they did have and make the best of their situation. They poured everything they could into the business to keep it afloat: all their energy, time, and almost all their money.

They found housing was their biggest expense by far and, whether they were renting a home or an apartment, the stress of maintaining consistency for their children seemed overwhelming.

One afternoon while Heather was on Pinterest, an online scrapbooking site, she saw a cute "pin," labeled "25 Campers You Have to See." She clicked on it with casual interest to see what people had done to design cute campers when something clicked inside her head. As she scrolled through the images of camper after camper she thought, "I could live here!"

A few years before, she and Graham had investigated the idea of a Tiny House, but to build a tiny house would take money upfront they didn't have, and building one was a bigger project than Graham had the time, energy, or experience to take on. But Heather felt that she was on to something with this cute camper idea.

She did a quick search through Craigslist and found a few RVs that seemed reasonable and in a size that could work for her family. She messaged her idea to Graham, and he thought it was genius. Within three days, Graham had taken action, selling his Jeep wrangler and using the money to buy and renovate a small RV, along with purchasing a used Tahoe to tow it. They were on the move!

Living in an RV isn't a conventional idea for a family of six, and at first it didn't make sense to some of their family and friends. Two hundred and thirty-two square feet isn't a lot of space, but what impressed me most when visiting was how efficiently it was organized. Everything had its place. From bunk beds and shelving for the kids' area to a cut-out for the cat to sleep under the kitchen bench, it was planned out with precision. Graham hired someone to help him with the updates they needed and learned along the way. Now he can make those improvements himself.

The biggest change for Heather and Graham wasn't in the space; it was in their housing expenses — reduced from over $2000 a month to under $550 for lot rent (the land where their RV sits) including water, electric, and sewer. They felt free.

Heather and Graham eventually decided to close their gym. It was a hard decision, but living in their tiny house gave them options they never would have had before. Graham was able to take a job as a caddy and work part time at Starbucks to pay their bills while going to school to learn computer coding. Just a few months later he was able to get an entry level coding job where he is learning more every day. This opportunity never would have happened if they hadn't C.H.A.S.E.D their Big Life.

First, they became clear about what they wanted and then created a plan with the small steps it would take to get there. They found the areas of their plan for which they needed to find help and the areas where they needed to attain more education. Then they started taking those steps. They regularly stop and examine where they are and re-evaluate their decisions for their future. Living small is their way of Living Big.

The Ripple Effect

Their decision has had a ripple effect on their families and friends. Heather's sister goes to college in North Carolina and works as an intern in the summer in Atlanta. She purchased her own little RV and rents a space a few doors up from Heather and Graham. This has given her the freedom to live on her own, not take on more debt while in college, and own something she can use later or gain some of her money back by selling. Living in an RV was an option she never would have thought of if not for Heather and Graham first taking the plunge. And Heather's mom, who recently went through a divorce, decided that tiny living is for her too.

What started as a solution to keep their business afloat became a calling, and Heather has now started a non-profit. "Tiny Beginnings: Fresh Starts for Families" is Heather's brainchild for helping families begin again. For $10,000 she can get someone an RV, renovate it, and provide a few months of lot rent. This could be a life-saver, keeping families together that otherwise may have succumbed to the stress of financial failure.

Starting small to Live Big has enabled Graham and Heather to create a life they couldn't have imagined before. Finding a calling and being able to help others is icing on the cake, and they feel stronger than ever as they move forward with their Tiny Beginnings dream.

Maybe, like Graham and Heather, Living Big for you means having housing without financial stress, and tiny homes would be a great option for you to investigate. Maybe Living Big is having a home in the mountains or at the beach, and starting small would be a way to achieve that. Thinking differently can lead to great solutions and can impact your life in positive ways.

Going Big in a Small Way

Lyndsey went against the grain and didn't listen to friends who thought she was crazy when she chose to buy a small condo in the late 90s. As a twenty-three-year-old who wanted to establish some consistency for herself, she took advantage of a special employer first-time forgivable loan and went to work finding a new home.

She found a 360-square-foot condo for $63,000 and was happy with her new place. It was easy to maintain and gave her the opportunity to have something of her own, which, at her age, was a great deal. She got some backlash from friends and family who didn't quite understand how buying such a small condo made sense, but Lyndsey always felt it was right. After living in her condo for about five years the real estate market crashed. Suddenly, having paid so much for such a small space seemed like a mistake after all, but Lyndsey saw it as an opportunity.

Many of the units in her building were going into foreclosure, and people were starting to sell at extremely low prices. She decided to take a risk and bought a 700-square-foot unit for $31,000. Again, people who love her were trying to protect her by telling her it was a mistake. The word was that real estate was never going to recover, and they feared Lyndsey was taking a risk that was too big.

The fact that Lyndsey knew what her larger goals were, was saving regularly with her company 401(k), and was buying places that cost much less than she could afford, gave her new choices. She could easily make decisions she thought would be best for her, so she ignored the naysayers and pushed forward.

Lyndsey told me, "People always need affordable places to live, and this was totally an affordable place!" She moved into the larger unit and rented out the smaller one to pay the mortgage.

Although being a landlord gets a bad rap, Lyndsey enjoys it. She takes great care of the condo she rents, screens people carefully, and her renters appreciate the great place they get to live. She's created a system that works for her and, in her small way, is building wealth.

A few years later, when Lyndsey decided to get married and buy a home, she rented out her larger condo and put all the additional income into principal payments so she could pay the loan off, creating more options for her new and growing family.

By taking small steps and not going too big from the start, Lyndsey created an environment she could grow with. Although real estate isn't for everyone, starting with 360 square feet allowed her to move up without feeling any extra pinch in her wallet and helped to ensure financial success down the road.

Roads Less Traveled

Both of these stories are important. Lyndsey's, because she took small steps to create a big future, and Heather and Graham's, because they recognized that going big too soon didn't work. They made adjustments and now are walking paths that can help others.

What about you? Maybe you are in living in the in-between — comfortable in your home, but not building wealth either. You don't have to walk down either of these roads to live a Big Life financially. Remember, it's about what's a Big Life for YOU.

There are lots of ways to Live Big while being financially sound. If you are trying to save money or get back on your feet, you don't have to stop having adventures or cut back on experiences. Adventures and experiences are what make life fun and help us create amazing memories.

There are some great sites online that offer information on house swapping if you want to go on an extended vacation and are on the adventurous side. These sites offer a new way to vacation and many have a vetting process to help you find the right match for your swap.

Try taking small trips instead of big vacations. A long weekend away can give you a needed time-out without breaking the bank. Driving somewhere you can get to in half a day can give you the feeling of having traveled, yet not so far away from home that you lose time driving. Small trips are some of my favorite memories of spontaneous weekends away!

Try a "staycation." Wherever you live, I guarantee there are things you haven't explored yet. Google "Cheap staycation ideas [Your city]" and see what pops up. If you want to be creative, grab your camera and go on a treasure hunt looking for cool landmarks and fun places to check out.

Looking for a weekend away with your honey but not sure what to do with the kids? Try switching weekend childcare with friends. If you don't have kids, but do have pets, you can share the load with fur babies too. Be creative in finding adventure and ways to Live Big on the cheap. Here are a few more:

- Go on a lunch date instead of a dinner date. Some acclaimed restaurants have lunch options that include smaller portions of their dinner menus for a fraction of the price. Save your wallet and your waist at the same time.
- Check out local parks and festivals. This is a great way to get outside and be part of something bigger without having to spend a dime.
- Check out Groupon or another online discount site for tickets to an event at a reduced rate.

There are loads of ways to Live Big on a budget. Being creative can be part of the process to living a Big Life now instead of waiting for later.

How will you C.H.A.S.E. your Big Financial Life?

CHAPTER 5

FINDING YOUR PASSION

Almost every successful person begins with two beliefs: the future can be better than the present, and I have the power to make it so. — David Brooks

We spend more time at work than any other place in our lives[1]. The average person reports spending 47 hours a week at work. That equates to six days a week. Compared to other countries, like Sweden, where workers put in an average of 31 hours, or Ireland where they work 29, the United States tops the list. On top of that, American work hours are on the rise. Nearly four out of every ten Americans work more than 50 hours a week.

The stress this can put on our lives and our families goes without saying, especially if you are doing work that has no meaning to you. Spending 50 hours a week doing something you don't enjoy has

---

[1] http://www.gallup.com/poll/175286/hour-workweek-actually-longer-seven-hours.aspx

a trickle-down effect. After a long day, it can be difficult to avoid letting that unhappiness seep into the other hours of the day. The hours spent with family and friends should be the most fulfilling parts of your life, but if you spend it complaining or worrying about work it can negatively impact every aspect of your life.

Of all the ways to die, do you know what can be predicted with a high degree of certainty?

A heart attack.

More heart attacks occur Monday morning between 5:00 and 10:00 a.m. than any other time of the week[2]. You know the drill: you live for Fridays; you watch the clock, drive home in a frenzy (with most car accidents happening during those evening commute hours); you dive into the weekend, but by Sunday afternoon, the dread is starting to creep in — you know tomorrow you have to go back to work and start the whole cycle all over again.

Doing work you love can improve your stress levels, your relationships with family members, and your health. It can lead to a Big Life. Are you living with a career that you love and inspires you? If not, do you wonder how to get from here to there? Developing a vision for your ideal day and then moving forward with the C.H.A.S.E. framework will give you structure as you press on to explore what it would mean to have a Big Life.

It's A Zig and A Zag

When I was growing up I wasn't one of those kids that just *knew* what they wanted to do. Some of my friends knew they wanted to be teachers or fireman, but I was never one of those kids. One of my friends even knew he wanted to be a mortician — and he is!

What I did know about myself was that I liked people. I liked meeting and connecting with new people during the day. I liked when friends came to me for advice or help figuring out a problem. After college, being in sales seemed like the best option for me. It

---

[2] http://www.drsinatra.com/heart-attack-risk-factors-rise-on-mondays/

wasn't the work I always wanted to do, because I really didn't know what I wanted to do, but I enjoyed people and liked the work enough to keep on doing it.

Back in college, I'd had an idea to open a personal training studio. I had always loved working out and felt like it provided a lot of benefits besides keeping me healthy. It was great for calming stress and also provided a social outlet. Opening a studio, I thought, would be a great way to do something I loved and work with people, which is what I felt like I was good at. All those years ago I looked into it, but I didn't have the capital or the knowledge, so I put that dream in a box on the shelf and went on building my sales career.

Then, 30 years later, I read a blog post about a woman who decided to go for her dreams later in life. I started thinking about it and got the idea to combine my love of helping people with fitness and bring boot camps to the park!

Why not?

I had a sales job where I traveled a lot, and the timing seemed right. My daughter was heading into the tween years, and I felt that I should be home more. So, I got a big van, had it wrapped in advertising of big pink kettle bells, and filled it up with gear. With the help of a few friends, I ran boot camps in the park that whole summer every morning at 5:00 a.m. After a month, we added evening classes, and I started to plan how to move out of my corporate job. We wore shirts that said, "We do it in the park," which felt creative and fun and unlike anything I could do in corporate America. I was taking the leap, and doing something I'd always wanted to do. Besides being fun, it let me try on my entrepreneurial spirit for size before tossing my corporate job to the side.

We eventually moved those boot camps to a retail location, opened up a CrossFit gym, and I left my full-time job to run the business. I needed a website, so I watched some YouTube videos on how to build one and, after some trial and error, created a website that was pretty awesome. Later, I was able to create the website that became betsypake.com.

A few years in, I talked to a woman who was in her 50's and had written a book. I decided I had knowledge and experience to share and that led me to write my first book, *Become A Nutrition Ninja*.

A year after that, I sold my gym. About the same time, I read Hal Elrod's *The Miracle Morning*, which started to change my mindset and helped me imagine new possibilities for my life. I took to heart the practice of getting up early and focusing on personal growth every day. I went to seminars, talked to people about what they were focused on, decided I wanted to be able to help more people live a Big Life, and began writing this book.

None of these events, by themselves, are particularly amazing, but they all added up to me taking control of living my Big Life. Taking one action opened my mind up to another. When I started the boot camps in the park, I never expected to be here, writing this book. It is never a straight line from one place to another. The line to achieving what we want is a zig and a zag. How could we know what it's like to run a small business if we've never run a small business? Trying one thing leads to the next. Experiences build to new experiences you don't expect at the onset, and getting started is the biggest key to moving forward.

If you've tried different jobs before, don't let that hold you back from trying something new. Everything you've done has been a step on the way to discovering where you want to be. Opening yourself up to new thoughts and ideas is a really small, yet smart, step toward understanding what your life's work could be.

Finding Your Calling

If you aren't Living Big in your career right now, maybe it's because you don't know what you want to do. It's time to spread out and explore, expose yourself to new ideas, find out what other people are doing, and discover what you love.

Start by pulling out the C.H.A.S.E. worksheet (or download a new one at www.StartSmallToLiveBig.com) At the top, write down where you are today in your career. At the bottom, write down where you want to be. That could be as simple as "find out what I want to do," or "discover my calling." Then, set your timer and begin brainstorming small steps you can take that will help you find work you love.

Here are a few ideas to get started:
- Read a book on a topic that interests you. The book doesn't have to be relevant to what you think you want to do; exposing yourself to different ideas can help you find new ways to move forward.
- Journal. Write every day. Focus on what you enjoyed during the day and what you can see yourself doing more of. Writing about the difficult parts of your day can also help you learn more about yourself and gain clarity.
- Share with others close to you about wanting to move toward a new career. They may have thoughts about ways you shine that you never thought could become a career.
- Set a timer and, on a separate sheet of paper, brainstorm for 10 minutes about activities you love. Don't stop until the timer goes off.
- Listen to podcasts. Be inspired by new ideas.
- If you have an idea about something you'd love to do, research it. Find out how others got started, and write down your own ideas about how to begin.
- When you find work you think you would love to do, volunteer in that field. It can help you meet people and discover whether it's really something you want to do with your life.
- Have adventures. Expose yourself to new cultures, new foods, new ideas. Trying things that make you feel alive and adventurous can help you determine what paths you should explore next.

When you discover a career that lights you up, follow the C.H.A.S.E. framework to bring that calling into life. Even if you aren't able to do what you love full time, working toward it can bring you peace, and being involved in the work can help increase the value you bring to the world.

Because They Love You

I have made a few transitions in my career and in my life, and so I speak from firsthand experience on this one: anytime you are changing your course, people close to you will be concerned. They will reach out and encourage you to go back to something "safe." They will tell you to do what you know, not what your soul calls for.

This, my friends, is because they love you.

They love you so much, they are scared for you. They don't want you to be in pain, and they don't want to see you fail. To the people who love you, it would be a safer bet to stay in the job you know than to risk trying something new.

Now I am not suggesting you drop your full-time, full-paying gig to jump into work you think lights your life on fire. I'm simply suggesting that as you start to move toward a life you love, people will get nervous. Ignore them. Be cautious for yourself, but ignore the naysayers that you love, and build toward the life *you* want. In the end, it is YOUR life and YOUR decision. In the end, it is YOU who will have to be okay with your choice to give it a go or take the safe route. Nobody else.

It's Never Too Late

Ellen DeGeneres wasn't always a comedian. In fact, she wasn't even known as "the funny one" in her family. Growing up, she wanted to be a veterinarian, but when that didn't pan out she worked waitress and secretarial jobs. One day, while giving a talk to her office, she found herself extra nervous. She used humor to overcome her nerves and when the group laughed, she lit up! She had found what made her feel purpose and happiness — she had found her calling. From there, she worked in small steps to make her dream of making people laugh every day a reality.

Maybe, like me, you grew up reading the *Little House on the Prairie* series. But you may not realize that Laura Ingalls Wilder didn't publish her first novel until she was 65 years' old. It's never too late to find what you love.

Takichiro Mori was an economics professor until he was 55, when he left to start a new business. He got involved in real estate first in his home country of Japan, buying up homes in the neighborhood where he grew up in Tokyo. When he died at age 88 he was a Forbes, two-time awarded World's Richest Man with a net worth of around $13 Billion.

Grandma Moses, one of the most celebrated names in American Folk art didn't start painting until she was well into her 80's. Even then, she started as a way to explore her passion for creating after her arthritis made it too difficult to continue doing needlepoint.

All of these people did work they loved and found their calling. You may be still in school or you may be 40 years into your career — it doesn't matter. You are able to do anything with your life that you desire, and there is *always* time.

If you are not on the risky side, finding your passion is still important. It doesn't mean you change a career, but perhaps add the work you love into your life in other ways. Bringing more meaning and happiness to your life is always good.

CHAPTER 6

BALANCED HEALTH FOR LIVING BIG

If it doesn't challenge you, it won't change you. — Fred DeVito

Health is about more than looking fit or being in shape. Being healthy is about feeling great. It's about having energy and feeling alive. It's about being able to do what you love to do without pain or limitation.

My friend Faigy lived a life like so many of us — with high stress and a never-ending to-do list. Taking care of her family came first and, with seven children, her own health was low on her list of priorities. She knew her diet suffered and she didn't take care of herself like she should, but Faigy didn't realize how off track she was until her mom got sick.

Faigy was in her 40's when her mom, one of those special moms who always went out of her way to make people feel welcome, became ill. She went into complete shock when her mom passed away suddenly just a few months later. Faigy had relied on her mother, and her passing left an enormous void in her life.

Within just a few months, Faigy began breaking out in rashes from head to toe. She didn't feel well and had no explanation for what was happening. She went to doctor after doctor, and they all were just as baffled. They asked if she had changed detergents or was using a different cleaning product in the home, but she hadn't and wasn't. They prescribed steroids and multiple rounds of antibiotics to try to identify and eradicate the source of the trouble, but none of it worked. The medication only seemed to make Faigy worse. The shock and stress of her mother's passing still fresh, Faigy decided it was time to stop all visits to the doctors and pay attention to her own body and nutrition to find the source.

She knew she was going to have to find her own answers. She searched the internet to find others who had experienced anything similar that would help shed light on her condition. After hours of investigation, she suspected that years of being nutritionally unbalanced, combined with the stress from dealing with her mother's death, had caused her immune system to shut down. She suspected she had "latent candida," an overgrowth of yeast.

Our bodies are truly miraculous, and when one system goes off kilter, they try to regain balance by altering other systems. The result of this balancing act created a domino effect inside Faigy's body, forcing her to change her nutrition drastically to begin clearing up the skin condition.

With dietary changes and months of focus, the rashes started to clear and she began feeling better. Taking control of her health, being an advocate for herself, and working to create a loving environment for her body helped it regain balance and get back on track.

You don't need to wait until you are feeling bad to start paying attention to your body. You can start implementing small changes now that will affect your health positively. Faigy's struggle has now become her calling, as Faigy shares her experiences with others online who are also searching for solutions.

Your Health-Limiting Beliefs

Most of us know that increasing the amount of unprocessed, whole foods in our diets can help us feel better, overcome long-term problems, and improve our waistlines but, in order to change, we have to stop the limiting stories we are telling ourselves. Having owned a CrossFit gym and coached people online, I can tell you that one of the biggest obstacles holding people back from achieving their Big Life in the area of health is their belief about what their bodies can and cannot do.

About a year ago I got a call from a friend of mine who wanted to talk about her weight. Mary had always wanted to be fitter and feel better. She'd tried many diets over the years, and each time she failed. She would lose some weight, but soon it would come creeping back, or she'd focus on a diet and gain weight within the first few weeks. To Mary, it seemed hopeless. I listened to her vent on the phone:

"I've never been one to lose weight easily. It's always been hard for me. My lifestyle just doesn't support me being the way I want, I guess. I feel like I have tried so many times…if it hasn't worked yet, it probably never will. My mother was the same way. I think I got it from her."

Remember what we learned about belief systems in chapter two? Mary was filled with self-limiting beliefs about her weight. Sure, there were strategies I could give Mary, and we'll talk about those in a minute, but nothing was going to help in the long term if she couldn't believe in herself.

How did I decide if Mary had real limitations or she just simply *thought* she had limitations? As a disclaimer, I will say that in rare cases there may be an undiagnosed, underlying medical condition that causes a client to fail to achieve weight loss and fitness goals but, in most cases, lack of progress is closely tied to beliefs about what's possible.

We can help Mary diagnose a helpful or non-helpful mindset by asking the simple question: Does this way of thinking help her reach her goals? If the answer is "no," then we need to find where she's limiting herself and determine a prescription for change. Let's break it down:

- *I've never been one to lose weight easily.* The Obvious. Mary has said this to herself so often it rolls right off her tongue. Does it help her reach her goals? No. She needs to shift.
- *My lifestyle just doesn't support me being the way I want, I guess.* The Sneaky. The "I guess" makes me believe that Mary didn't realize this was how she felt. This one slipped out, indicating that, deep down, Mary believes her lifestyle could be what's holding her back. She's unsure if she's even in control.
- *I have tried so many times…if it hasn't worked yet, it probably never will work. My mother was the same way. I think I got it from her."* This is a classic Hand-Me-Down. So often we take on the beliefs of those who are closest to us. Losing weight was hard for Mary's mother and Mary saw her struggle. Her mother was either on a diet, coming off a diet, or about to go on a diet. So Mary unknowingly thought adult women should live their lives that way.

Once we see where Mary is holding herself back, it's important to help her create shifts that support her goals. For Mary, having a Big Life includes being carefree and happy in her body. This is the process I followed to help her create new beliefs that support her goals.

She and I talked about how she imagined it would feel to be a comfortable weight.

"What would that type of person, the person who is thin and 'put together' be like?" I asked her.

Mary described what that type of person would be like — slowly at first, and then, as her picture became clearer, more detailed. That person, "...would be able to go out with friends and not feel like she had to eat everything on her plate. She would stop eating when she started to feel full. She would like to exercise and move her body every day. She would look good in clothes, and it would be effortless to put together an outfit that worked and she felt confident in." As we continued the exercise, Mary's tone changed. It was fun to hear her get excited about how great that person would be who was all that Mary wanted to do and be. I knew she had a clear vision, but she didn't believe it could be a vision of herself.

"So what," I asked her, "would be different in this person from what you told me about yourself? What beliefs would you need to adjust?"

As we talked, Mary began identifying the beliefs she needed to shift and poking holes in what she believed was possible for her life.

The first was believing she could lose weight. She knew her body was capable. She had lost weight in the past and recalled those times.

When I asked her what someone who loses weight easily is like, she decided it was someone who exercises as part of her life — as something she loves to do. She went on to explain, "That person probably likes fruits and vegetables." She got really clear about what that person was like!

Think about your own journey and any struggles you have had with fitness and health. Do you limit yourself in your thinking? Becoming clear on what you want and then imagining a person who lives the life you want is an incredible exercise for any area of your life. Once you have an idea of the habits that person would have, you can start to incorporate those habits into your life too.

Use the C.H.A.S.E. framework to get clear on where you are headed.

But what if you have no idea? What if you don't have a clear idea of what a healthy person does regularly? What if you aren't sure how to model them because you aren't familiar with the choices they make every day? Research. The internet is a fabulous tool, because you can find out more about any sort of people you want to meet.

You can learn about their habits, plug into groups they are in on social media, and ask questions. Soon, you'll have answers, and you can begin to model those behaviors too.

So what does someone that is healthy do? I have some simple strategies that will help you get moving in the right direction, and the great thing about these strategies is that they all start small.

I'm going to share a few anchor habits you can get started on to increase your energy and get your weight in check. Some of these habits may seem odd. They may be new to you. Choose the ones that work well in your life and remember to start small: making one of these a habit before moving on to the next will help you incorporate these habits firmly into your life. They will become a part of who you are — a healthy person.

Anchor Habit #1: Eat Slowly

Do you remember when you were learning to drive a car? Your parents probably enrolled you in a drivers' education course and then prayed to the insurance gods that you were safe and wouldn't have an accident. And what was the one thing your mother would say right before you drove on your own the first few times?

"Don't drive too fast! Be careful!"

That's because she knew that more speed meant less control.

It might be eating out with friends or watching TV while you are at the dinner table that causes you to eat a little extra, but speed and distractions can be a deadly combination when it comes to your waistline.

I feel the need...the need for speed – Maverick, in Top Gun

Have you ever come home from work, totally stressed and exhausted, knowing you have to start making dinner, but there's a bag of chips on the counter and you figure you need a minute to catch your breath, so you grab the bag, throw yourself down on the couch, and mindlessly turn on the TV? Handful after handful of chips go down before you reach the bottom of the bag and realize you hardly noticed you were eating.

We've all done that.

Here's where you use your new habit of eating slowly. Anytime you feel like you are starting to eat and cannot stop, or any time you are out with friends, or any time you normally have no control over what is happening, *slow down*. Eat what you want. Order what you want. But eat it SLOWLY. Remember, more speed equals less control.

What *is* "eating slowly?"

Eating slowly is taking a bite and chewing it all the way. It's relaxing between bites and not putting more food on your fork until you're ready for the next bite. Try putting your hands on your lap between bites. Take some sips of water. Talk with your family or friends. Then, take the next bite.

In the beginning, it may be helpful to set a timer. Wait 60 seconds from one bite to the next. Then after a few meals, lower it to 30 seconds and see what you can learn about your habits and your unconscious reactions while you are at the dinner table. Notice when it's harder or easier. Compare when you eat out to when you eat at home.

Many people who start this habit are surprised by how fast they normally eat, because they never gave it much thought. Doing the opposite of what you've always done is a great way to mix things up and start to notice deeply ingrained habits.

When you eat slowly, you notice more things about your food and how it effects your body. How it effects your mood! And how it nourishes you.

I'm going to be honest. There are times where I've rolled this habit out to my coaching clients and they get *real* fidgety. They paid to lose weight, not for someone to tell them to simply eat slower!

Learning to eat slowly is an incredibly effective anchor habit you can come back to each time you need to regroup or feel yourself getting off track. It is transformative. So trust me when I say, "This won't be an easy one! This may actually be one of the hardest habits to stick with."

There is one thing I know, from experience: food isn't just to nourish my body. It's emotional too! Eating quickly and denying yourself that emotional connection to your food and what it's doing for you only leaves you needing more. You can't rush through your meal and truly appreciate or get what you need from it.

When we start to feel nourished and emotionally fed, do you know what else happens? We find we don't need to "feed" in other ways, trying to fill our needs by:
- Choosing bad relationships.
- Accepting "less than."
- Shopping.

Shopping is actually a lot like over eating. We have an emotional need, we consume beyond what we need, and then we experience the guilt and shame cycle that goes along with it. Slowing down, being mindful, and having a *true emotional connection* to what you are eating can help in lots of areas. Where else can you see this habit of eating slowly helping?

Stacking

When you've successfully established one habit, begin working on the next habit. This method of "stacking" is a small change that will greatly increase the possibility of your sticking with the program and achieving sustainable changes in your health.

I had a client who called me for help a while back. I'd known her for a few years and really liked her, so I was excited to be working with her. We emailed back and forth and then decided to hammer out the details of how I could help her reach her goals. We set a time to meet and she decided right after work was best. She would call me on her way home, before she picked up her kids and life took over.

When the phone rang, she was super excited. I was happy to have a client so gung-ho and ready to get to work! And then it happened.

The list.

She had a list of things she wanted to get started on RIGHT AWAY. No waiting! She was ready!

The list ranged from cutting out all carbs (gasp!) to eliminating her four-times-a-day Mountain Dew habit. Oh, and she wanted to quit smoking. "Let's start first thing in the morning," she said.

"Ummm…" I looked nervously around the room.

You get it, right? We can't change everything all at once. It just doesn't work that way. Change one thing, make it stick, and then add on the next thing. Keep change simple and consistent and you will have success.

You don't have to be Superwoman or Superman!

I promise that is NOT how this works.

So, what does work?

Stacking. Just like we've been doing. Get in the habit of changing one thing and then stacking on the next.

Anchor Habit #2: Stop Eating When You Are 80% Full

Choose a day to start, and at every meal, stop eating when you are 80% full.

How will you know you are at 80%? If you have established anchor habit #1, you are eating slowly enough that you'll notice. (Pretty cool trick, eh?)

Seriously though, what *is* 80% full?

Remember a family celebration meal where you went to your grandma's or to your favorite restaurant and ate everything you wanted? That is stuffed. That's stuffed full — I'd say 120%, depending on how well your family cooks — unbutton-your-pants stuffed.

Contrast that stuffed feeling with what super hungry feels like — when your stomach is so empty you feel light-headed and a little sick. Let's call that 0%.

So where does 80% live? Somewhere in the middle. It's the point where you are satisfied but not stuffed, and not hungry anymore either. It's the point where you could keep eating, but you really don't need to.

So how do you find it?

If you are eating slowly, and you are paying attention, being mindful and enjoying your food, you'll start to figure it out. Maybe not at the first meal, but you'll discover your 80%, if you:

- Slow down and pay attention to how your belly feels.
- Use a smaller plate and/or leave some food on your plate and see how that feels.
- Stop, give yourself a break (try five minutes) and see if you are still hungry enough to keep eating. Remember: don't starve yourself. Just stop a little bit earlier.
- Be patient. You don't have to be perfect.

If you have been following along and working on these habits, you may be wondering when you will start losing some weight. You've been sticking to your new habits and eating slowly. You're doing the opposite of what you used to do, so why isn't the opposite happening!

There is a lot changing under the hood.

You may have heard the story about the farmer and the bamboo:

A farmer worked his land and did all the necessary steps to prepare his land for his Chinese bamboo seed. He carefully watered and fertilized it every day, but at the end of the first year, nothing happened. The bamboo didn't even begin to sprout. The farmer had faith and so he continued to work. The second year he watered and fertilized the seed every single day, but at the end of that year, there was nothing. The third year, nothing. The fourth year, still no growth at all. The bamboo didn't show any signs of growth for four solid years. But the farmer continued his practice of watering and fertilizing what he had planted. Then the fifth year came. The Chinese bamboo

> shot up at an unbelievable rate, and in a matter of just six weeks, the bamboo hovered at 90 feet tall.

Bamboo grows *down*, beneath the surface for years before you can actually see the stalks. Bamboo grows so tall that if it didn't first grow down and create those strong roots it would never be able to maintain its growth and height.

Right now, you are working on fertilizing your soil.

Changes ARE happening, although you may not see them yet. You may be feeling different. You may be thinking differently. Know that long-term changes aren't always seen on the outside, but once they are, they are much stronger and more sustainable than they would have been otherwise.

Anchor Habit #3: Eat Lean Protein At Every Meal

Lean protein can help you get lean and assist you to stop eating when you are 80% full. This habit is pretty simple: simply add lean protein to every meal. Lean protein includes:
- Wild game
- Lean beef
- Poultry (chicken or turkey
- Fish or seafood
- Eggs
- Protein powders
- Tofu or Tempeh
- Dairy, such as Greek yogurt or cottage cheese

As you start adding more lean protein into your diet, you may have more energy, feel full quicker or stay full longer, and start to lean out. Our bodies need protein to function properly, and many times we just aren't eating enough of it.

Eating and digesting protein takes work and your body will burn more calories dealing with the increase in protein than it will with carbohydrates or fat. This extra work will keep you full longer and help you to maintain the anchor habit of stopping when you are 80% full.

Anchor Habit #4: Eat Veggies At Every Meal

Eating a serving of fresh vegetables or fruit at every meal can help you feel full, increase fiber in your diet, and give you increased energy. Vegetables add bulk to your meals without adding a lot of extra calories, and they are almost always fat-free.

A lot of people don't like vegetables, and that's why they stay away from them. If that describes you, chances are you haven't seen all the different sources of veggies and fruits available to you. There are different ways to prepare them, and different varieties to try, so if you feel like you aren't on the vegetable train just yet, that's okay. Do the opposite of what you've always done and branch out.

- Hit up a farmers' market and see what's new and local. Locally grown fruits and vegetables can taste a lot better than what you get at the grocery store and that has traveled a long way to get to you.
- Try a co-op that delivers fresh local food to your doorstep. They usually don't allow too much substitution, which gives you a chance to try something you never would have bought at the grocery store, and they will often include new recipes for the vegetables in the box.
- Fruit can be an awesome alternative to a typical fat-filled desert. Trying new fruit can be fun and interesting too!

Keep in mind that your focus should be on vegetables, as they are less calorie dense than fruit. Although fruit is natural and healthy, it usually holds more calories per serving than vegetables. Shoot for five servings every day, each portion about the size of your closed fist. This small habit can have a huge impact on your health, and you'll find yourself looking forward to adding those veggies to every meal.

Anchor Habit #5: Move Your Body

We are often under the impression that to have a huge impact on our health we need to make massive changes. But the truth is, even with exercise, small steps are more manageable and giant leaps can do more harm than good.

A 2011 study[3] found you can actually slow down aging and add an additional three to seven years to your life by doing one simple thing every day: exercising. The study found that exercise significantly increases an enzyme that helps repair your DNA and these benefits can be seen in only six months. Simply adding 25 minutes of cardiovascular activity daily could change your life expectancy and halve your risk of heart attacks in your 50's and 60's. Amazing results for such a small change.

In addition, regular movement, even as simple as walking, has been shown to lessen depression, anxiety, stress, and even calm ADHD symptoms[4]. If you've never exercised, remember starting small is perfect. Starting small is starting where you are *right now*.

About a year ago I got an email from a woman who wanted me to help design a new exercise program for her. The problem, as she described it, was that she had zero time during the week. Her only time was on the weekend, so she wanted an intense exercise program created for two days a week. She was fairly new to exercise, so I wondered about her joints and muscles. Would it damage her body to engage in this kind of intense exercise? Would she be so sore on Monday that she would be discouraged from starting again when the next weekend came around?

With all these questions rolling around in my mind, I decided to ask if she had time to get up 15 minutes earlier every weekday. She did, and so we put together a program in which she walked for ten minutes every morning before she showered. Just ten minutes — simple enough —but that gave her 50 minutes of extra cardio during

---

[3] https://www.ncbi.nlm.nih.gov/pmc/articles/PMC3320801/

[4] http://pediatrics.aappublications.org/content/134/4/e1063.full#sec-8

the week. Hardly even a blip out of her schedule, yet she could cut her weekend workouts in half and still get the same amount of overall exercise time. On top of that, she would be creating the habit of moving her body every day while protecting her joints from overuse. Starting small was definitely a way for her to Live Big!

Don't underestimate having just five or ten minutes a day to work on a C.H.A.S.E. step or task. Ten minutes a day is five hours over the course of a month. Imagine if you increased your movement by five hours this month! How different might you feel? Do you think it would make a shift in your motivation, in your clothes, and in your energy level? Absolutely.

C.H.A.S.E. Healthy Habits

Remember, you cure lack of motivation by getting into action. Think super small and be creative in ways you can work toward eating better and incorporating movement into your life.

Can you feel the difference in starting small as compared to starting out the first day trying to do everything at once? You'd never have day two! Start small and build on each success.

CHAPTER 7

THE VALUE OF TRUE CONNECTION

The meaning of life is to find your gift. The purpose of life is to give it away. — *David Viscott*

Whether it's in our careers or in our personal lives one fact stands clear: genuine success can't be reached without spending time focusing on building great relationships. Relationships are the heartbeat of everything we do and the foundation for everything we want to build in the future. But we live in a culture where our view of achievement and success focuses on career and money. When all our efforts are flowing toward one area of our lives, the remaining areas tend to suffer. To live a Big Life we need to find balance. I believe that spending time on relationships is spending time in the right place.

What would having great relationships do for your life? Not only your relationship with a partner, but also with your children, friends, relatives, and co-workers? How would your life change if you knew how to make these relationships thrive? If you don't have warm, interesting, comforting relationships now, how is this lack causing you to suffer?

Rat Park

Jonathan Hari gives an incredible TED talk[5] where he explains the importance of connecting with people in relationship to the problem of addiction. He tells of an experiment conducted in the 1970's by a group of professors at Simon Fraser University. They observed that when a rat in a box was given two types of water, one regular and one laced with heroin, the rat would always choose the water with the drug in it. Over and over again, rat after rat, they recorded the same results. Drugs must be addicting, at least in rats, and the researchers concluded that fact probably translated to humans as well.

The group of professors noticed that all the experiments were with one rat on its own. They were curious and, to try something different, designed a "rat heaven." They created a large rat enclosure they called "Rat Park," which included tunnels and color boards and lots of other rats. There were lots of activities for the rats inside this enclosure and, most importantly, they had companionship.

The professors found that the rats that had lots of interaction, found partners, had babies, and were social didn't drink the heroin water. The single, caged rats overdosed almost 100% of the time, while the rats in Rat Park had an overdose rate of 0%.

This study got Jonathan Hari thinking. Could it be that our addictions to food, shopping, drugs, and even to work, are fueled by our lack of connection? Could relationships with others fill the innate human need to connect and help us overcome those additions? Could our lives be easier, and could we gain control of those behaviors that seem to control us by simply focusing on building ties in our lives?

---

[5] https://www.youtube.com/watch?v=PY9DcIMGxMs

Even if you don't suffer from a drug addiction, or get cold sweats when you have to turn your cell phone off, or eat to feed your feelings, or feel the need for "retail therapy" you can't afford, you may be surprised to find how much your relationships influence your happiness. Having close bonds and connections can make a difference in virtually every area of your life. As you continue to think about how to C.H.A.S.E. your Big Life, don't underestimate the power that relationships have on your success.

Focusing on the right things.

I sat at brunch with my friend Christy. I'd known her for longer than I'd known my husband. Craig and I had met at No Excuses CrossFit five years before and been married just over a year. I was frustrated.

Sitting in that restaurant, over flavored coffee creamer and eggs benedict, I complained to Christy, "I'm just not sure Craig and I are on the same path."

Before Craig, I had been single for seven years, since Olive was four, and marriage was an adjustment. I was used to making all my own decisions. Learning how to cooperate with someone else was a struggle.

Christy looked me straight in the face, and in her Alabama accent said, "All that talk about opposites attract just ain't true. You need to get to the bottom of the story — and that's that you and Craig share the same values. You both believe in honesty and truth and hard work. All that other stuff is just stuff. Stop worrying about it." With that, she went back to eating her English muffin.

This was so simple, yet made so much sense. When it comes down to it, we don't want to spend time with people who are totally different from us. We want to spend time with people who are similar and share the same values. Whether Craig likes one political candidate and I like another doesn't matter as much as the fact that we both believe in honesty, trust, and integrity in our lives. I needed to stop looking for the cracks — the differences — and start noticing where we were alike.

This small shift had a tremendous impact on how I approached everything moving forward. In disagreements, I began looking for our commonality. In discussions about our finances, I tried to understand where we thought alike and then build on those agreements. We share experiences, and these experiences bring us together.

The truth is, what you focus on is what you are going to see. Just as my friend Kyle actively focuses on what he can accomplish instead of any excuses he may have, the same philosophy can be used with our relationships. Focus on unity, shared values, and the stories you share. Build upon those things. We all have more in common than you might think — it all depends on where you are focused.

Family Matters

Gary Vaynerchuck, entrepreneur, author, and internet personality, starts his morning with a routine that includes relationships. Gary is someone who has built an incredible empire in business, and thrives on "the hustle," so I was surprised to discover that he focuses each morning on family. Each day, when he drives to his office, he calls his mom, dad, or sister, depending on which one he called last. He does this to simply catch up and as a reminder that their relationship is important to him. He does this to connect. These don't have to be big long conversations; in fact, because he does it regularly, catching up doesn't take very long. Like Gary, working time to connect into your routine can help even the busiest of us create the relationships we want. It's a small change that can have a big impact.

If you want to follow Gary's example, and the idea of making these calls stresses you, start small and proceed step by step. Start by simply programming the numbers into your cell phone. Next, put them on your favorites list. Then schedule a time to call one person each day. Set an alarm to remind you to make the call. Finally, make one call. If you already have great relationships with everyone in your life, calling someone every day may seem over the top, but if you don't, and your "flight or fight" response is triggered by thinking about starting this practice, start small. Ridiculously small.

Big Relationships

Creating a Big Life — in all areas of your life — means taking time to decide what kinds of relationships you want.

I have learned that small, consistent actions matter more than big, once-in-a-blue-moon actions. If I take a minute each day when my husband comes home from work to look in his eyes, ask how his day was, get out of my technology (put down my cell phone) and into the moment, magic happens. When I slow down and express genuine interest in what someone else is interested in, I begin to understand that person better. I see how others' experiences have brought them to where they are in life and how much they have to share.

Mahatma Gandhi suggested that we "be the change we want to see in the world." I think there is no place where that is more true than in our own homes. Become the partner you are looking for. Work on yourself first.

We can't change others; we can only change ourselves.

When I become the partner I want to have, I notice my partner works to do the same. When people feel heard and understood, when they feel you are trying, it's easier for them to try, too.

Listening To What Isn't Said

My eleven-year-old daughter lay on the floor in my home office. Something wasn't right and I'd known it for months. I just could not put my finger on it although I'd tried.

She didn't talk much. She rolled around, first staring at the ceiling and then rolling onto her side to face my desk. I had always felt we were close, but mother-daughter relationships can be strained, and we had hard times in the past.

She turned to look at me as I was about to walk out of the room, and I caught a glimpse of truth on her face. I felt as if I were seeing her for the first time. I saw her as a stranger would see her. Lying there, looking at me, all so obvious.

It was like when someone walks in your home and you see it through their eyes. You look around the house and notice all the things that didn't stand out before. You see the stack of books on the table and the breakfast dishes still on the counter top. You realize it's more "lived in" than you would like a stranger to see.

Just a few minutes before, I hadn't noticed anything out of the ordinary, but now…now I saw my daughter as though through a stranger's eyes, and it was all so clear I was surprised I hadn't noticed it before.

"Do you like girls?" I asked her as she lay motionless on the floor.

She sat up, looked at me, with both a pained and relieved expression on her face, and then anguish took over.

"I don't want to!" her little voice broke.

I'm grateful my reaction was slow. Methodical. I already knew exactly what I wanted her to understand from my reaction: love. And so it was simple for me. No big outburst or confusion. I was clear. She was clear.

I sat on the floor. We talked. We made plans. How do we tell people? When do we tell them? Who do we tell? We ordered rainbow flags from eBay. And we hugged. A lot. (If ever you have the opportunity to show your child what you really meant when you said, "I'll love you no matter what," take it.)

And moments of silence were okay. Understanding that silence was okay when Olive and I talked was a big change for us. In the past, she would speak, and I would immediately think I needed to respond and give her the answer. I'm the mom, after all! I should be able to help. But realizing that kids (and adults too) don't always need a solution, that they just need to be heard, allowed me to slow down and pay attention to what she was saying. I could let it settle in, and then, if there was something I didn't understand, I could ask questions and go from there.

When I listened in this way, I could see when she was feeling uncomfortable by how she moved her body, if she wouldn't look at me, or if her eyes had tears. When I stopped trying to problem-solve and started listening, our communication grew.

I haven't always done things right when it comes to relationships. In fact, if you were to look at my track record, you'd say that I have probably fallen on the side of failure more often than not. Relationships are complex and wonderful and not always easy to navigate. But I found that failing can lead to some pretty great insights, if you're paying attention.

I've discovered we need to listen. And not just to the things that are being said, but also to the things we notice but nobody talks about. We need the courage to ask questions when we don't understand, and when the answers aren't clear, to ask more.

I've learned that we all need to be cheered on. To be told we are worthy and amazing. Capable of everything we could ever dream. We need others to believe in us when we fail to believe in ourselves. We need connection.

There will be all kinds of relationships in your life. Some will begin and some will end; others will change and grow with you. Forming bonds with people is critical to your happiness. But don't confuse social media and online connection for the kind of connection you need. When you have a crisis or need a friend, chances are you can't reach out to someone you just met on the internet.

Take the time to form those important relationship bonds. Discuss your beliefs around connection with people who are important to you and see what you need to change within yourself. Find places to connect in real life and people who are seeking the same values and experiences in relationships that you are. Search for what you have in common, even with those you have the most difficult time getting along with, and listen to the unspoken words.

C.H.A.S.E. relationships that matter and sustain you.

CHAPTER 8

OUR COMMON THREAD

When you are broken, you run. But you don't always run away. Sometimes, helplessly, you run towards. — Helen Macdonald

Years ago, I heard a parable about Buddha that I've never forgotten:

> A woman in a small fishing village had lost her only son to an illness that took him unexpectedly. In her grief, she went to Buddha and begged him to bring her boy back to life. He told her he would create the medicine necessary to complete such a task if she could get a mustard seed from anyone in the village whose family had not been struck by grief.
>
> She ran from house to house, asking if anyone could help her. Although everyone wanted to provide comfort and give her the mustard seed she so desperately wanted, not one could say that their family had been safe from grief and mourning.

> *Stuck, the woman realized she was not alone in her suffering. She buried her son and went to the Buddha to tell him she was unable to fulfill his request. She gained some peace knowing that death was a part of life that she shared with everyone else in the village.*

If you only associate living a Big Life with always being happy, you are missing out on so much opportunity to grow. Suffering makes us who we are, makes us understand each other, and makes us learn more about ourselves. Suffering is as much of living as being happy. I believe it makes us more human by increasing our capacity to love and have empathy for others who have experienced loss too.

In order for us to live a Big Life, we must change. And with change comes loss in some form or another. Loss can leave us feeling isolated and confused, but there is something there for us in those desperate times that can help us grow. If we learn to use the experiences of grief, failure, and loss as tools to better understand what we want in our lives and what is important to us, suffering becomes valuable. Our need for connection is especially strong when we feel most vulnerable. When it comes to loss and grief, we all have something to share.

My Story

I was a junior in high school and my sister Amy was a sophomore in college when she and my mother decided to head out of town for a hockey game at the university my sister attended. It was a few states over but my mom was spontaneous and fun, so when they decided one night they would leave the next morning, I wasn't surprised.

On the way there, they got lost and, in trying to find her way back to the main road, my mom lost control of the car and was killed. From that point on, the lives of everyone in my family changed. It altered how I saw the world and provided me with a viewpoint different from any of my friends at the time. Life can change in an instant and never be the same again.

What I remember most about that time wasn't hearing the news of my mom's death as much as all the support we received from friends and family: the cards and sweet notes I got at school, and people acknowledging what had happened when they saw me instead of ignoring it or pretending everything was the same.

Small Starts

Space. Allow yourself the space to mourn for as long as you need to. You may be grieving over a death or another type of loss, such as realizing your dream has changed, or your life has turned out differently than you expected it to. The idea of extended mourning can feel uncomfortable, because who wants to feel bad? We want to take our mind off things and to be happy. But ignoring your feelings when you are grieving any sort of loss will make things much harder in the years ahead. Grief will bubble up when you don't expect it, making you feel out of control. Remember, it's okay if you feel like you have to cry. It's okay to laugh. It's okay to continue on living and having emotions of your own. I have found that letting myself experience the emotion is better for my healing than trying to push it away. Experience your different moods however they come to you. If you are supporting someone who is grieving, his or her mood may change from one moment to the next. Go with it. Let it be and just know that being there makes a difference in that person's life.

Connection. If you are the one grieving, people may not know what to say or do. They want to help but don't know how. Tell them! Don't be afraid to ask for what you need. You may need to talk out your thoughts and emotions or you may just need to have someone sit with you. Having meaningful connections is important, so let friends know what you need. If you tend to isolate yourself, find ways to reach out and connect with a supportive group. A small step in that direction may help you feel better and lead to other opportunities to be around people who understand your struggle.

Choice. After my mother died there were many benchmarks in my life along the way that made me angry. I was angry I didn't have my mom to share in the experiences and lean on when I needed guidance. What I realized in these times was that I had a choice: I could choose to be angry and put my life on pause or I could keep going, searching for the lessons I was supposed to learn and finding the small gifts along the way. Staying open helped me find nuggets I felt were lessons sent from my mom, which brought me comfort.

Help. Volunteer to help someone else. One thing we all share, as shown in the mustard seed story, is this experience of loss and grief. When you reach out to help someone, either by volunteering or getting active in your community or church, you feel a sense of purpose and belonging you may not have felt since your loss. You also meet people and find you share that common bond. Helping others can help you see that others have gone through what you are going through, and who have grown in the process. You may be encouraged by their strength and realize you may have strength of your own that you didn't recognize before this experience.

Mindfulness. Connect with yourself every day. Use meditation, visualization or even art or exercise. It's important to take care of yourself when grieving. Imagine that grieving is like running a marathon. If you don't take gel packs, stop occasionally, and get help bandaging your feet, it will be a long, uncomfortable road. But if you take care of yourself, the journey will be less painful. Find yourself in art or yoga, doing something with your body that takes your head out of the grieving space. When we have unprocessed feelings, engaging the creative side of our brain can help us start to connect with ourselves and find who we are again after a loss.

Starting small will help when you are dealing with loss and death. Ordinary daily activities may seem more difficult than they did before. Don't put pressure on yourself to keep everything the same as it was before, because everything probably seems different.

Remember that the key to overcoming any obstacle is breaking it down into those small steps that are achievable for where you are in your life right then. You don't have to pretend everything is the same as it was, and you don't need to apologize for feeling different about things that brought you joy before.

Decide now what would make today a Big Life and C.H.A.S.E. that day until the next day when you break it down again. Step by step, your Big Life will come back into focus and you will create your new normal for your future.

CHAPTER 9

THE BIG KAHUNA

Everything in life is a vibration. — Albert Einstein

I believe, and you may agree with me, that living a Big Life includes spirituality — an area of life that connects you to something bigger than yourself. This may take the form of a religion you have grown up and are comfortable with, or it may simply be a realization that you can connect with a larger energy through another path, such as nature or art.

My spiritual path has changed throughout my life, and what I found to be true for me evolved as I learned more about myself. But at the root of it all was the belief that there was more to life than just me and that being connected to this energy was important for me to live a balanced life. In my journey, it became less about which religion was "right" or "wrong" and more about what made me feel most connected, where I found meaning, and how I wanted to share the world with others.

Reconnect with Your Spirituality

If you are like me, you may have gotten disconnected from your Big Spiritual Life by getting bogged down with "everyday life." This sense of disconnection is something I hear from a lot of people. If you've been put off by organized religion in some way, that doesn't mean you can't begin to find a connection to something outside yourself. One way to begin is to do more of what you love. Reconnect with activities you enjoyed in the past. You don't need to start a big project; just incorporate some of those activities into your daily life — they will reinvigorate you.

If you can't remember what you loved, grab a blank piece of paper and a pen and set a timer for five minutes. Start the timer and then start free-writing about what activities bring you back to a feeling of being centered, when you feel most like yourself, or things you did in the past that helped you feel calmed and refreshed. List whatever comes into your mind. Open up to what brings you joy and what you loved to do as a younger person. Using the timer pushes you to keep writing past the surface ideas and get into your subconscious.

When we are doing things that bring us joy, we are more connected to ourselves and can find that inner spirituality that brings us peace.

Meditation

Here are a few small actions you can take to connect with your inner spirituality. As the popularity of yoga and mindfulness have come in vogue, it's not surprising to hear so much talk about meditation too. What has been surprising to me is the number of high powered executives and CEO's of all faiths who have turned to meditation as a regular part of their busy schedules.

Meditation is known to control stress, battle anxiety, lower blood pressure, help your immune system and even help you reach your goals. With all those great benefits, it sounds like a magic pill, and I think it might be. Large companies, like Aetna, Apple,

Google, and Proctor & Gamble are taking notice and incorporating meditation into their strategy for employee health, offering midday meditation classes for employees.

If these large companies are pouring resources into this practice, maybe it's time to slow down and take a closer look. I started my meditation practice just a few years ago, and at first it was a real struggle. My mind is very busy and I found myself overwhelmed. I started by trying to sit in meditation that first day for 20 minutes, my mind swirling. It didn't take longer than one session like that for me to remember to start small, so the next day I sat for five minutes. Soon I was up to 10 and then 12 minutes. Now I sit, some days, for close to 45 minutes in meditation, and I've found I look forward to it so much that on particularly stressful days I go back for a second round before bed.

The greatest thing about meditation is that it is impossible to worry when you are meditating. Mindfulness and meditation mean being fully present in the moment. Since stress is simply thinking about something in the future and being unsure how it will turn out, when you are focused on the moment you are in, there can be no cause for worry or stress. Meditation helps reframe where you are and brings you back to that connection with your spirit.

Getting Started

The whole idea is to just get settled. Sit in a comfortable chair and focus on your breathing. You don't need anything fancy, no "tools" other than your breath. I started out sitting for just five minutes. That's it — five minutes of sitting and focusing on my breathing, in and out. Big deep breaths and pushing the air out. This is called *Mindful Meditation,* and here are some recommendations to help you get started:
- If meditating in the morning doesn't work for you, use the time you have available. Maybe it's lunchtime or before bed. Be fluid and fit it in when it works for you.

- I found at first it was really hard to "not think." I kept thinking..._I'm not supposed to be thinking._ And that was thinking, so not really helpful. Know that it's okay to have thoughts come into your mind. Just let them come and go. Don't follow them down the road to wherever they are going. Your mind will start to quiet itself, but it won't happen right away. Be patient and don't be worried about doing it wrong.
- Imagine a golden light coming down from the sky, through the top of your head, down through your chair and back up again. Doing this gives your brain something to focus on. When I do this, I imagine the light matches my breath, breathing in when the light comes down and exhaling as it goes out into the sky. This helps me focus and be aware of where I am in that moment.
- Another way to quiet your mind is to use a mantra. A mantra is simply a word or a sound that is used during meditation to help you concentrate. I found a video on YouTube that I think sounds really beautiful of chanting Tibetan monks, but you could use a recording of ocean waves or the sound of birds. Some people chant "Om" or "One," which I think is a great way to keep your mind from wandering. Try some different techniques and see what works for you.
- Try a guided meditation. This can help you work through anything from mindfulness, to focusing on a goal, to releasing fear or being more creative. There are many guided meditation apps you can download to your phone. I like one called Omvana. A great meditation to start with is the Six-Phase Meditation by Vishen Lakhiani, and it's free on Omvana. This will guide you through mindfulness, being present, and visualizing your future.

With daily meditation practice I feel so much more awake and alive, my heart is open to people, and I find I don't get nearly as distracted by that voice in my head. I am able to focus on specific areas of my life, and find an inner calm that helps me feel more balanced.

Practicing Gratitude

I had a friend in college who wanted a Volkswagen bus. It was the early 90s and they weren't manufactured anymore, but she seemed to see them everywhere she went: parked on the side of the road, on someone's tee shirt, or on a TV show. Those buses were everywhere, and she spotted them!

That's how it is with gratitude too. Once you decide to be grateful, you begin seeing things to be grateful for. You start to notice what has meaning and value for you. Even when life goes wrong, you are able to pick out a nugget of happiness, because you've trained your brain to be on the lookout.

Here are two simple ways to train your mind, create a gratefulness practice, and put the universe on notice that you are ready to manifest some greatness through gratitude.

- Each morning, write down three things or people you are grateful for before you start your day. For me, it's simple things, like cuddling with my dog first thing in the morning, or appreciating the morning light that comes in through my kitchen window. These stand out in my mind because they are everyday things. Life doesn't have to hand you incredible life-changing, monumental events for you to find gratitude. The best way to retrain your mind is to recognize gratitude for the simple things. Learning to appreciate those small things helps create your Big Life.
- Use the *Five-Minute Journal* to develop a gratitude practice. You can buy a hard copy of the book or the app. I've used both. Using the *Journal*, every morning my daughter and I each write three things we are grateful for, three things that would make the day great, and decide on an affirmation for the day. At night, we finish our day by writing three things

that happened that we are grateful for and one way we could make tomorrow better. In this way, even on the worst of days, I find myself easily able to find a nugget of happiness.

Volunteering

Volunteering is not only a great way to feel connected to our communities but also a way for many of us to increase our satisfaction with our own lives and feel like we can serve a higher purpose. If you have spent some time focusing on what would make your life more complete, you may have noticed that connection continues to rise to the top. For many of us, feeling grounded in relationships and community makes all the other successes that much more satisfying. Volunteering is a way to add a selfless component to your spiritual practice and allows you to share your gifts with someone else.

My sister, Amy, has always made a practice of volunteering for a cause she believes in. As kids she would join 24-hour "rockathons," where kids would gather to raise money for a particular cause. She was always the one volunteering to pick up trash in the community on "Green Up Day," and she was always the one looking for ways to bring attention to something she thought was important. So it's not surprising that she continued on that path as an adult, currently working with a non-profit in her city of Seattle.

Amy serves on the board for the Mockingbird Society. It's an organization that works to end youth homelessness and improve foster care. Amy is not from Seattle but has a wide range of friends in the area because she followed her passions to serve. Her connection to that community is deep. She moved from Nashville to Seattle ten years ago, and I had seen her do the same in Nashville — finding ways to get involved in a cause that meant something to her.

Doing good is good for the world, but doing for others will also make you feel like you have more time not less[6]. It connects you to the community and helps you make an impact.

---

[6]   https://hbr.org/2012/09/youll-feel-less-rushed-if-you-give-time-away

Amy has given countless hours over the course of her lifetime, but she probably wouldn't explain it that way. According to studies on volunteers, people who volunteer, want to give even more[7]. They are more willing to give more time and money toward causes that are important to them. Volunteering gives Amy energy and connection, and she feels purpose and value when sharing her time.

Volunteering can help give legs to your spiritual practice and it's simple to get started. Almost any cause needs help or support in some way. It may be with an organized volunteer effort or simply to help in their office. Search out a cause you are passionate about and check their website for volunteer opportunities.

In larger cities, you can check out organizations like Hands On that will match you with different volunteer opportunities, so you can try them out and see what interests you. Habitat for Humanity has many home building sites across the United States you can get involved in.

If you are up for adventure, there are volunteer vacations available in locations all over the globe. You could do good, see a different part of the world from the community side instead of the tourist side, and create a memory you'll never forget. You can find volunteer vacation options online or check with a travel agent to be sure you are going to a safe place with a well-respected travel company.

Finding yourself in spirituality most often means finding importance outside yourself. When we connect with what is larger than ourselves, our lives take on more meaning. No matter your cause, you can always find a way to plug in and connect. Shifting your focus to something outside yourself can help you C.H.A.S.E. that Big Life by helping someone else live theirs. Get out your worksheet right now and see how your Big Life unfolds when you introduce spirituality into your vision. Can you work in any of the small practices that have been mentioned, or can you think of other small steps of your own?

---

[7] https://nonprofitquarterly.org/2015/01/28/must-read-fidelity-study-on-link-dynamics-between-giving-and-volunteering/

CHAPTER 10

THE POWER OF STARTING SMALL

I hope by now you are beginning to understand the power of starting small and have used the C.H.A.S.E. framework to create ideas for ways to start living your Big Life. If you're excited about achieving your Big Life, that's great, and why I wrote this book. But being excited isn't enough. We have to get into action. We have to begin doing those small steps that move us toward the lives we are destined to have.

The ways to incorporate small steps into your life are endless and where you start depends on where you want to focus. It all begins with taking just one action. Any action. If you've done a C.H.A.S.E. exercise, pick one small step you can do daily. Find one that is so small it would be silly to skip it. Consider starting with an action that takes under five minutes to accomplish. Perform that action consistently, and then build on it. You can choose to focus on any area of your life. The trick is to just get started. Once the ball is rolling you may be surprised how quickly these small steps pick up momentum and create a big impact on your life.

Rocket Ships

At the beginning of every school year, my mom would encourage me to start off the year with a big push by reminding me that a rocket ship uses 80% of its fuel to get off the ground. If I could manage to stay focused in the beginning of the year, then I would have more success later on. She was hoping that success would propel me into action! She was right. A slow start made for a slow year but if I could manage to stay engaged and focused those first few months, the rest of the year went much smoother.

Many times we wish for motivation and wonder how others have the energy to do what they do, but the reality is that motivation doesn't come before action. Action comes first, and motivation is built through its progress. When you begin with one step, no matter how small, you are setting the wheels in motion and motivation is not far behind.

Once you have momentum toward your Big Life, it will become easier and easier to keep the ball rolling. Accomplishing one small task every day toward your goal will establish habits that create your Big Life.

Take the pledge now to have awareness around your daily actions and direct them in a way that builds toward the life of your dreams.

The Breakfast of Successful CEOs

There are lots of small ways we can improve ourselves, but a way that really works for me is incorporating a morning routine. Over and over again we hear that the most successful CEOs have consistent morning routines that allow them time to work on themselves every day. They create time before everyone else is up to improve themselves, have time for breakfast with their families, and still be at work by 8:00 a.m.

Oprah meditates 20 minutes each morning. Arianna Huffington describes her mornings as most joyful when she incorporates yoga and meditation. By 5:30 a.m., Starbucks CEO, Howard Schultz, is exercising with his wife. These highly successful people all know that morning is best to create time for yourself.

Before you disregard this idea completely, remember — small steps. You don't have to get up tomorrow morning at 5:30 a.m. when you are used to getting up at 7:00. Rising only ten minutes earlier than usual would allow you close to an hour of self-improvement time in a work week. Ten minutes a day allows enough time to read about 10-15 pages of an inspiring book that could help you think differently and learn something new. That's 105 pages a week, 420 pages a month, or two books. If you were reading 24 books a year, do you think that would have an impact on your growth? You bet it would!

When we get started, it's normal to feel an extra surge of energy. Our vision is clear, maybe for the first time in years, and we are ready to make things happen. It's exciting, and so, when we start to feel down or discouraged about our progress we may begin to wonder if we've lost our drive or if we are not "good enough" to have success. Those times will come. It's normal, and there are things you can do to get yourself back into the groove.

Change Your Focus

In 1993 Jimmy Johnson was the coach of the Dallas Cowboys as they were headed to the super bowl. He knew they could win if they had focus. In the locker room he prepared the team for the game ahead, reminding them of the importance of focus. He told them, "If I put a 2x4 on the floor right here and told you to walk across it, you would all make it. But If I put that 2x4 up, 10 stories high, between two buildings, only a few of you would make it across. Why? Because your focus would be on falling, not on walking across the board. You must focus on the right things as we play this game!"

When does your focus move toward what you don't want instead of what you do want? When do you get down or feel discouraged? Do you know how to change your thought processes so you are focused on the good that you want for your life? If you are struggling with this, head back to chapter 2 and review the process to make that shift. Because once you figure out what your Big Life is, hard times will come. Struggles will come, and you will need to be ready if you're going to get past them.

The Secret of Shifters

Music is a big mood shifter for most people. Hearing a song on the radio can immediately bring you back to a time in your life when you felt happy and joyful. Hearing music that inspires and makes your soul move can allow you to imagine success in your mind's eye, as well as make other concerns seem less important.

Create a song list containing songs that improve your mood and increase your sense of happiness. When you need to shift your focus, put on a song and let it take you away for a few minutes. Regroup, get back into action, and move forward.

As part of my morning routine, I play a song I like, and I (literally) jump around the room, getting excited about the day ahead. This practice makes a huge difference and helps me to start the day focusing on abundance and moving forward in my life.

Amy Cuddy, author of *Presence*, shares the power of how body language changes your brain chemistry. It turns out that jumping around the house with my hands in the air to make me feel powerful is rooted in science! Moving my body actually helps to lower my cortisol and increase my testosterone. These are two key elements found in most powerful leaders; testosterone aids in confidence, and lower cortisol helps to decrease anxiety. Standing in a "power pose," (think Superwoman or Superman) for only two minutes can help shift your hormones — and makes you feel great! Try to be in a bad mood standing with your hands in the air listening to some great music. It just won't happen.

Visualize

I also use visualization as an active part of my morning routine. After I wrote my perfect day, as described in Chapter 2, I began reading it every day. I would imagine my day, using motivational music in the background (check out movie soundtracks for some great visualization sounds!) and feeling it as if it were real. Having this vision helped create a blueprint for my mind's eye. As I went through my day, I would notice things that I may have passed by before, things that could help me on my journey to fulfill that vision of how I wanted to live my life. If I'd never had the vision, and reminded myself of it daily, I may have missed some clues along the path that would help me live my Big Life.

I read about a study in which athletes had been divided into three groups. One group practiced free throws, a second group only visualized the free throws, and the third group both visualized and practiced. It's no surprise to me that there was no difference in performance between the group that visualized and the group that physically practiced.

You can't do anything if you don't imagine it in your mind first. So, creating your perfect day and regularly visualizing it will train your brain to understand the outcome you are looking for.

Take the 30-day C.H.A.S.E. Your Big Life Challenge

If reading this book has inspired you to take action, then don't wait. Get started right now. Make the commitment to start Living Big today. That means there is something better out there for you and that you are ready to go get it! Waiting to Live Big or for something to magically happen doesn't work, so now is the time to make a plan and get going.

You can accomplish more than you ever dreamed possible for your life.

I invite you to embark on a 30-day challenge. Taking this leap will build momentum, and results will come faster than you imagined.

Begin this 30-day journey of action, and when YOU start to change, everything around you will be transformed as well.

To join the challenge, head to www.StartSmallToLiveBig.com and sign up for the free challenge, where you'll get access to trackers, downloadable resources, and helpful lessons along the way.

One Last thing

Two things I know to be true: learning without action is useless and hard things are easier with friends. If you got something out of this book, if it altered your thinking or inspired you in some way, I'd like to ask a favor.

Ask your friends to read it. Let them know what could be possible and let them know that you believe in their Big Life. We all need someone to believe in us and we all need help along the way.

Howard Thurman said, "Don't ask yourself **what the world needs**. Ask yourself what makes you **come alive**, and go do that, because **what the world needs is people who have come alive**."

We need you out here. We need them. Spread the word and let's do this together.

RESOURCES

Below you will find links to people mentioned in the book and the C.H.A.S.E. worksheet. Download these worksheets and join the challenge at www.StartSmallToLiveBig.com

Faigy changed her eating to regain her health. You can find out more at her website Live Better With Faigy: http://www.healingnaturallywithfaigy.com/

Kyle Maynard opened the CrossFit gym where I met him and learned more about changing our beliefs to better support our goals. You can find Kyle at http://kyle-maynard.com/

My sister Amy volunteers at this great organization that helps improve foster care and end youth homelessness. The organization I talked about is The Mockingbird Society and you can find it at http://www.mockingbirdsociety.org/

Rene Godefroy is an inspiration to many. Born in a small Haitian village, he changed his circumstances to live a life where no condition is permanent. You can find out more about Rene here http://www.renegodefroy.com/

Lyndsey made sacrifices in her housing with a goal of freedom. She now runs an organization helping others quit their day jobs and start something of their own. You can find her at www.QuittingCorporate.com

C.H.A.S.E YOUR BIG LIFE
Create. Help. Attain. Start. Evaluate.

Where are you now? What do you want to change?

10 Minute Brainstorm:

Continue on back ->

Vision of where you want to go:

Step 1: Write out the problem & what you want to change. At the bottom of the page, write out what Living Big would mean to you in the context of this problem. Set a 10 minute timer. In the middle, write out all the small steps you could do that would take you toward that vision. Don't censor it. Just write.
Step 2: Find areas you need to get help to move forward and circle those things.
Step 3: Find where you need to learn or get something else to be able to move forward.
Step 4: Get started! Put a box around a few things that would have the biggest impact and put them in your calendar.
Step 5: Evaluate weekly. Before you week starts, sit down and determine what needs adjusting and what is working. Add new small tasks to your calendar.

CPSIA information can be obtained
at www.ICGtesting.com
Printed in the USA
FSOW02n1441070217
30501FS